Vic   JAN 0 4 2011

D0470734

616.342 BAR 2010

Master Your IBS :
An 8-week Plan to Control the

Master Your IBS

An 8-Week Plan to Control the Symptoms of Irritable Bowel Syndrome

Pamela Barney, MN, ARNP
Pamela Weisman, MN, ARNP
Monica Jarrett, PhD, RN
Rona L. Levy, MSW, PhD, MPH
Margaret Heitkemper, PhD, RN

VICTORVILLE CITY LIBRARY
15011 Circle Dr
Victorville, CA 92395
760-245-4222

Master Your IBS

AGA Institute Publications Committee

Sheila E. Crowe, MD, AGAF, Chairman

J. Sumner Bell III, MD, AGAF   Fred S. Gorelick, MD

Anthony J. Lembo, MD   Cynthia M. Yoshida, MD, AGAF

AGA Press Advisory Board

Colin W. Howden, MD, AGAF, Chairman   Lawrence J. Brandt, MD, AGAF

Rick Davis, Jr., PA-C   Melinda Dennis, MS, RD, LDN

Steven Flamm, MD   Daniel A. Leffler, MD, MS

David C. Metz, MD, AGAF   Melissa Palmer, MD

Amy Shaheen, MD   Helen M. Shields, MD, AGAF

AGA Press

Christine B. Charlip	Division Director of Publications
Sherrye Landrum	Book Editor
Circle Graphics, Inc.	Design and Composition
McNaughton & Gunn, Inc.	Printing

Disclaimer

This publication provides accurate information on the subject matter covered. The publisher is not providing legal, medical, or other professional services. Reference herein to any specific commercial products, procedures, or services by trade name, trademark, manufacturer, or otherwise does not constitute or imply endorsement, recommendation, or favored status by the AGA Institute. The views and opinions of the author(s) expressed in this publication do not necessarily state or reflect those of the AGA Institute, and they shall not be used to advertise or endorse a product.

©2010 by University of Washington. All rights reserved. No part of this book may be reproduced or utilized in any form or by any means, electronic or mechanical, including photocopying and recording or by any information storage and retrieval system without permission in writing from the publisher.

ISBN 978-1-60356-009-2

Printed in the United States of America   13 12 11 10   1 2 3 4 5 6

Library of Congress Cataloging-in-Publication Data

Master your IBS : an 8-week plan to control the symptoms of irritable bowel syndrome / Pamela Barney ... [et al.].
   p. ; cm.
   ISBN 978-1-60356-009-2
   1. Irritable colon—Popular works. I. Barney, Pamela.
   [DNLM: 1. Irritable Bowel Syndrome—therapy—Popular Works. WI 113]
   RC862.I77M28 2010
   616.3′42—dc22

           2010037832

For additional copies or information on licensing or translating this content, please contact:

AGA Press
4930 Del Ray Avenue
Bethesda, MD 20814-2513
www.MasterYourIBS.com

A PROGRAM OF
THE AGA INSTITUTE

Contents

WEEK 5

WEEK 6

Acknowledgments

Many people helped make the production of *Master Your IBS* possible. We thank Linda Burton; Barbara Glenn, RN-C; Gaile Moe, PhD, RD; Bruce Naliboff, PhD; Susan Nivert, MN, ARNP; and Sheldon Rosen, MD.

Thanks to Michael Camilleri, MD, AGAF; Lin Chang, MD, AGAF; and William Whitehead, PhD, AGAF, for their review and constructive comments. We are also indebted to Christine Charlip, AGA Press, for her editorial and publishing expertise.

The book is based on research supported by the National Institute of Nursing through National Institutes of Health grant R01NR004142.

About the Authors

All five authors work at the University of Washington, Seattle.

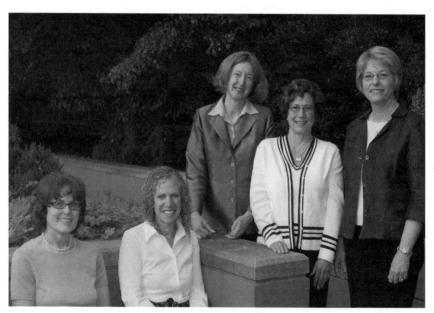

Left to right, Dr. Jarrett, Dr. Levy, Dr. Heitkemper, Ms. Weisman, and Ms. Barney. Photo by Gavin W Sisk, UW Creative.

Pamela Barney, MN, ARNP, an adult psychiatric nurse practitioner, has worked for many years in the School of Nursing on NIH-funded research with a focus on the management of IBS symptoms. She played an active role in designing and implementing the self-management treatment used in these studies. As a clinician in private practice, her work focuses on self-management of stress-related illnesses, including IBS, headaches, fibromyalgia, and chronic fatigue as well as the treatment of mood disorders, anxiety, and sleep disorders.

Pamela Weisman, MN, ARNP, is an adult psychiatric nurse practitioner who specializes in self-management therapy for a variety of disorders, including IBS, anxiety, depression, and insomnia. As a clinician and a research nurse at the School of Nursing, she has been a member of numerous nationally funded studies that focused on several self-management strategies presented in this book. Ms. Weisman's expertise is stress management, biofeedback, and relaxation training.

Monica Jarrett, PhD, RN, is a Professor in the Department of Biobehavioral Nursing and Health Systems whose research focuses on functional GI disorders in women and men. Dr. Jarrett is directing three scientific studies (two in women and one in men) that explore potential physiological and psychological causes and/or factors that exacerbate symptoms of IBS.

Rona L. Levy, MSW, PhD, MPH, FACG, AGAF, a psychologist and social worker, is an expert on the psychological aspects of functional GI disorders such as IBS. She was central in the development of the protocol that served as the basis for *Master Your IBS*. Dr. Levy is Professor of Social Work, Adjunct Professor of Medicine and Psychology, and Director, Behavioral Medicine Research Group, University of Washington. Her research on factors associated with functional GI disorders and intervention strategies to reduce their impact is funded by several NIH grants.

Margaret Heitkemper, PhD, RN, FAAN, is the principal investigator of the National Institutes of Health–National Institute of Nursing Research study from which this program was developed. She is Professor and Chairperson, Department of Biobehavioral Nursing and Health Systems, and Adjunct Professor, Division of Gastroenterology at the School of Medicine. Her NIH-funded research focuses on women's health, gender, and sleep disturbances.

To the many people with irritable bowel syndrome who have shared their time, their stories, and their knowledge to help us better understand effective methods of managing IBS symptoms.

You Can Master Your IBS Symptoms

Maria had a reason for wanting to get her irritable bowel syndrome (IBS) symptoms under control. Although she had been bothered by IBS since childhood, her abdominal pain, cramping, and diarrhea were now significantly interfering with her life. For years she had dreamed of starting her own catering business. Working toward that goal, she signed up for a new cooking class that would help fine-tune her culinary skills. The class met weekly. Each person brought a different dish, and together they enjoyed a wonderful gourmet dinner. The class was filled with creative cooks, some of whom had professional experience, so each week Maria was amazed and sometimes intimidated by the dishes they prepared and shared. After the dinners, Maria's symptoms went into high gear and sometimes she even had to leave early and missed the discussions. She was beginning to dread each upcoming cooking class and wondered about her ability to actually make the catering business that she had dreamed of for so long a reality.

After considerable thought, Maria decided that she didn't want to give up on her dream. Instead, she would learn some symptom management strategies. Her physician told Maria about the ongoing IBS symptoms study at the University of Washington. This 8-week education course offered her the opportunity to learn new ways to deal with her IBS.

Maria attended the education sessions each week and worked patiently and methodically on incorporating the techniques she was learning into each day. She was introduced to a variety of strategies, including relaxation exercises that fit into her busy life, how to identify trigger foods, and ways to change her eating patterns. The program encouraged her to examine her thought patterns and consider new, healthy ways of thinking that worked for her. Of course, any lifelong pattern is difficult to break, and Maria encountered some challenges, with relapses into old patterns. But eventually, over time,

Maria was able to put together a plan that helped her effectively manage her IBS symptoms.

For nearly two decades, the University of Washington "Nursing Management of IBS: Improving Outcomes" study has worked with more than 300 people with IBS who, like Maria, desired to lessen the burden that IBS puts on their everyday lives. *Master Your IBS* presents the week-by-week techniques used in the Nursing Management of IBS: Improving Outcomes study that has helped so many learn how to manage their IBS symptoms and achieve greater freedom from IBS. The book is designed for you to read one or more chapters each week for 8 weeks. Each chapter provides an opportunity to learn new strategies for symptom management. Each week ends with a suggested homework assignment that encourages you to practice the new self-management techniques throughout the week. This week-by-week approach gives you time to understand the information, master the strategies, and incorporate them into your life. The strategies focus on awareness of diet, relaxation, and healthy thought patterns, and through them, you will come to better understand your IBS. Because every strategy does not help everyone in the same way, it is important to practice each strategy, evaluate its effectiveness, and like Maria, create your own unique plan that works for you.

Maria started by learning and practicing deep breathing exercises. She tried to practice these skills regularly throughout her day. Sometimes she remembered to do this, and sometimes she forgot. She worked to set up a reminder system, which helped her practices be more consistent. Soon she began to notice how much more relaxed she felt throughout the week. One of Maria's surprises was her new awareness of the large amount of time she spent worrying about the pain she might experience after her cooking class. Because she was committed to learning to manage her symptoms, Maria knew that she would need to change her thinking. Slowly, she made small changes. She worked on worrying less and considered the idea that she might be able to alter the outcome of the evening by changing how she thought about it.

Over several weeks, Maria crafted a plan to manage her IBS symptoms. It was a detailed plan that focused on ways she could relax, promote healthy thought patterns, and make a few simple dietary changes. She worked at each part of the plan throughout the week, practicing being aware of her feelings and stress levels. For each challenge that arose, Maria had to "play detective" to sort out the source of the problem. For example, she realized that the day of her class was often a busy and stressful day. By the time she arrived for class, she was hungry and exhausted. This gave her another specific behavior goal: figure out how to reduce her hunger and exhaustion. And Maria was impatient. She wanted instant change! Because this program helped her realize how her thoughts might increase her stress, she eventually came to see how her impatience was also part of the problem.

After several months, Maria realized that abdominal pain was no longer her primary concern, and she was having diarrhea less and less. When she did experience diarrhea, she realized that she had a new attitude about it and saw it as a temporary inconvenience, versus a daily fact of life. This helped her feel better throughout the week and increased her confidence that she would soon be able to open her catering business.

This book comes with tools that will help you reach your goal. It's important for you to monitor your symptoms using the Keeping Track forms in the Appendix of this book. We introduce them and explain how to use them in specific chapters, and there are extras in the Appendix that you can use in the book or copy. As you track your symptoms over an 8-week period, you will be able to see your progress and identify the strategies that are working for you. You will also want to use the Food Journal (there are extra blank forms in the Appendix) at specific points during the 8 weeks to help you identify the diet adjustments that you need to make.

During Week 8 there is an opportunity to review the strategies and develop a personal plan for managing your symptoms. At this point, you will have a clear idea about which strategies have made a critical difference in your symptom management and will help you master your IBS. Using the strategies that have been the most helpful, you will be able to write an effective symptom management plan. An effective plan is realistic for your life, specific in the amount and frequency that you use the strategies, and written in a measurable way so that it is easy to see when your goal has been met.

After Maria worked through the material in this book, she was able to write a plan that reduced her symptoms significantly.

Maria's Plan for Symptom Management

Relaxation

- Practice abdominal breathing exercises 4 times a day.
- Increase abdominal breathing exercises to once an hour on the day of the cooking class.
- Do a progressive relaxation exercise the morning of class.
- Get at least 8 hours of sleep the night before the class.

Thought Patterns

- Identify my "overgeneralization" thought patterns and change them to more accurate healthy thoughts as soon as possible.
- Avoid "fortune telling." Remember that there is no way that I can know how the evening will turn out. I have more control if I relax and let go of the worry.

Diet

- Eat every 3 to 4 hours.
- Avoid trigger foods (coffee, orange juice, broccoli, and high-fat foods) prior to class.
- Don't go to class hungry.
- Take a low-fat dish that is free of trigger foods to class.
- Have a low-fat snack before going to class.
- Eat small servings at dinner. Don't overeat.

Eight months later, Maria is attending an advanced cooking class each week and seldom has symptoms following the dinners. She has a plan for her catering business and hopes to open it within the next year.

Are you ready to learn skills that will help you recognize triggers and decrease symptoms? Read each chapter slowly, and practice the techniques on a regular basis each week. Some are as simple as taking a few minutes for yourself, to slow down and breathe quietly. You will want to understand and master each strategy so you can get the maximum benefit. Therefore, you may want to work on certain chapters for longer than a week.

Although some of the skills may sound familiar, we encourage you to practice each one several times. There is a difference in knowing the material and applying it to your life. Slow, structured practice at using these skills can make a welcome difference in gaining control over your IBS symptoms.

A New Approach to Irritable Bowel Syndrome

IN THIS CHAPTER

Learn about irritable bowel syndrome (IBS).

Understand how this new approach to IBS symptom management works.

QUICK FACTS

The cause of IBS is not completely understood. Three major factors influence IBS symptoms: altered bowel motility (the natural rhythm of the smooth muscle of the intestine as it works to move digesting food through it), increased intestinal sensitivity, and a disruption in the communication between your brain and gut.

The primary symptoms of IBS are abdominal pain relieved by a bowel movement and a change in the frequency or form of the stool.

Triggers can increase the frequency and severity of IBS symptoms. Common triggers are diet, stress, and negative thought patterns.

What Is Irritable Bowel Syndrome?

Irritable bowel syndrome is a common digestive disorder that affects both men and women. Approximately 10–20% of the population has symptoms compatible with the diagnosis of IBS. People with IBS experience a variety of symptoms

Criteria for IBS include abdominal pain or discomfort and at least two of the following:

- Pain that is relieved or lessened by a bowel movement
- Pain that is associated with a change in the frequency of stools
- Pain that is associated with a change in the consistency of stools

From Drossman DA. The functional gastrointestinal disorders and the ROME III process. *Gastroenterology* 2006;130(5):1377–90.

that vary from person to person and from day to day. Symptoms are varying combinations of abdominal pain, diarrhea (frequent or loose stools), constipation (infrequent or hard stools), gas, bloating, urgency, and mucus in their stools. Many have found that stress and certain foods make their symptoms worse.

You may be troubled with frequent bowel movements or frequent loose stools, for example, three episodes in the morning and another bowel movement after each meal. Stool may be watery or loose. Diarrhea often brings with it a feeling of urgency, and you need to find a bathroom—now. Or you may be troubled by constipation, with infrequent hard stools and need to strain while trying to have a bowel movement. You may have a combination of both problems.

Celeste, 21, has had a "sensitive stomach" since she was a little girl. As a child, she just assumed that everyone experienced abdominal pain, urgency, and 3 to 6 bowel movements each day, just like her. In college, the diarrhea and urgency became more severe, prompting Celeste to make an appointment with her doctor. After a complete evaluation, she was diagnosed with IBS.

Carla, 37, was recently diagnosed with IBS also. She suffers from severe abdominal pain and constipation. At times she will go several days without having a bowel movement. The pain can become excruciating, at times so bad that she has to stay home.

Brian, 53, manages a tire store and has had IBS for several years. His symptoms vary, without any apparent reason. He will suffer with abdominal pain, diarrhea, gas, and bloating for several months. Then, unexpectedly, his symptoms will change to pain and constipation. Several times he has suffered from pain, urgency, and multiple loose stools in the morning and hard painful stools in the afternoon.

Each of these people has different symptom patterns, but they all have IBS. Although their symptoms vary, IBS seems to rule their lives. They make important decisions about life based on the severity and frequency of these symptoms.

What Causes IBS Symptoms?

Although the cause of IBS is not fully known, research suggests that there are three major factors that influence IBS symptoms. These include

- altered gastrointestinal motor activity (called *bowel motility*)
- increased sensitivity to gut stimuli
- a disruption in the hormonal and nervous communication between the brain and the gut

Bowel motility is the process of the smooth (involuntary) muscle moving food and waste products through the intestines. The strength of the muscle contractions moving these materials and the speed with which these materials are moved through the intestine both influence IBS symptoms. For example, when food and waste are moved too quickly through the gut, you may have diarrhea. When the gut moves food and waste too slowly, this allows time for too much liquid to be absorbed, and hard, dry, infrequent stools (constipation) result.

Increased sensitivity to gut stimuli refers to the attention, perception, and meaning that people with IBS attach to any activity within the abdominal cavity. These sensations may include gas, bloating, gurgling sounds, cramping, left-sided discomfort, sensations of fullness or incomplete evacuation, or even having a bowel movement. People without IBS generally pay very little attention to these sensations. Those with IBS are usually very aware of the sensations as well as the anticipation of these sensations. Experiencing or anticipating these sensations activates parts of the brain that cause people to process them as negative, bad, or painful.

The brain and the gut send messages back and forth all the time. These messages are sent through the nervous system and influence bowel motility, release of digestive hormones and other secretions, and sensitivity as well as recognition and interpretation of gut activity. When there is a problem with the communication between the gut and the brain, these functions can be altered, for example, gut sensitivity or the perception of pain may be increased.

These factors can be influenced by several additional issues in a person's life. Stress, for example, can affect the network of nerves that carries messages between the gut and the brain. Relaxation, on the other hand, can help bring the nerves back to a more normal state. Diet, thought patterns, the location and amount of bacteria in the intestine, abuse, trauma, genetics, and hormones each have the potential to play a role in creating IBS symptoms.

For example, Shelly, 33, was consistently bothered by abdominal cramping and diarrhea and occasional constipation (altered motility). She had a demanding job that she was able to handle most of the time. But when deadlines approached, she struggled to get everything done. Her boss had a volatile temper and often yelled and made insulting comments to his staff. Shelly lived in fear of those outbursts. In fact, when she knew the deadlines were approaching, she was aware of every little gurgle and movement of gas in her intestine (increased sensitivity). As the deadlines got closer and her boss became increasingly anxious, Shelly developed severe diarrhea and spent much of the day in the bathroom (influence from the brain-gut connection).

During normal digestion, the food and fluids we ingest mix with enzymes that the body produces to break down the food into small pieces. The pieces then move gradually through the small and large intestine. As they pass along, water and nutrients are removed to feed our bodies. Fiber and other indigestible parts of food continue on to be excreted as stool. If the intestines move food along too quickly, not enough water is absorbed by the bowel, and the stool becomes soft or even liquid. This creates diarrhea. If the bowel processes food too slowly, too much water is removed, and the stool becomes hard and difficult to pass. This creates constipation. Anything that disrupts the natural rhythm of the smooth muscle of the intestine and the speed with which it moves digesting food through it changes how the bowel functions and may cause pain.

IBS Requires Self-Management

IBS is not life threatening, and the symptoms do not cause serious damage to your body. Having IBS does not increase your risk of developing other diseases of the intestines, such as cancer. Although some medications may help you manage your symptoms, they don't work consistently for everyone. Although, we don't know how to cure IBS, and it generally does not go away on its own, it's typical for the frequency and intensity to vary often over a lifetime. Symptoms may increase during times of stress, during different points in a woman's menstrual cycle, and when you don't get enough sleep. Symptoms often decrease during more relaxed times, when you are eating a healthy diet, and often during pregnancy.

Betty is a good example of how symptoms can vary over time. She is 60 years old and has had IBS for 45 years. She first struggled with diarrhea and cramping throughout middle school and high school. In college, she attended a competitive nursing school. During those years, her symptoms increased to the point that she considered dropping out of college. But Betty was able to continue and graduate. She took the summer after graduation off and her symptoms decreased significantly. The next fall she began her first nursing job, on the night shift. The work stress was high, and she had difficulty sleeping during the day. Again, her symptoms became severe. Two years later, Betty married Carl. She transferred to the day shift and decreased her work hours to half time; gradually, her symptoms decreased. Betty and Carl had three children. During her first two pregnancies, Betty was virtually symptom free. But in her third pregnancy, the symptoms increased once again.

Over the next few years, Betty's symptoms varied with stress, rest, and her menstrual cycle. After having three children, Betty decided that she wanted to lose the 15 pounds that she had gained during her pregnancies. She joined a weight loss organization that stressed eating small, well-balanced meals and exercise. Betty recalls that during this time her symptoms were almost gone entirely. Recently, Betty and Carl have retired. Their stress is minimal and they have time to enjoy hobbies and grandchildren. Betty is happy that once again the symptoms have decreased, and most days she can forget about having IBS.

IBS symptoms are distressing, uncomfortable, and inconvenient, and they may determine how you spend your days. Many of the participants in our study found that they were able to gain a sense of control over their symptoms as they learned new strategies and identified effective ways to incorporate them into their everyday lives. To minimize the disruption caused by IBS, you can learn to manage your symptoms and master your IBS.

What's Involved in Proper IBS Diagnosis?

A diagnosis of IBS from your health care provider has several parts. You told your health care provider about your symptoms, and they were typical of IBS. Your health care provider wanted to know how long you'd had the symptoms, when they occurred and what helped the symptoms or made them worse.

You may have had blood tests to check your red and white blood cell counts and electrolytes (such as sodium and potassium levels), a stool sample to check for infection. You may have had other tests done as well. Many people see a gastroenterologist for a sigmoidoscopy or colonoscopy to examine their rectum or large intestine.

With this information, your health care provider ruled out other more serious problems, like inflammation of the colon (colitis), parasites, or cancer. Your diagnosis came only when your symptoms, history, and other tests showed no other cause for your symptoms.

When to Consult Your Health Care Professional

IBS is not a life-threatening illness, and generally IBS symptoms can be controlled with self-management strategies. However, it's possible for your symptoms to indicate a more serious condition. It is important to contact your health care provider if the location, character, or severity of any of your symptoms changes.

For example, if you generally experience pain in the lower left side of your abdomen, and you develop pain in the upper right side of your abdomen, this is a change in the location of your pain. If your IBS symptoms usually include cramping abdominal pain, and you develop a burning sensation in your upper abdomen, that is a change in the character of your pain. A change from diarrhea to constipation that you have not experienced in the past is another change in the character of your symptoms. If your pain, diarrhea, or constipation becomes significantly worse, you have a change in the severity of your symptoms. If any of these problems happen, it's important that you follow up with your health care provider to rule out any additional problems.

Bleeding is not a symptom of IBS. If you have been diagnosed with hemorrhoids, you may sometimes have bright red blood with your stools. Do not assume, however, that if you have bleeding you have hemorrhoids. It is important to get unexplained bleeding checked by your health care provider and have your provider make the diagnosis.

If you develop a fever in connection with your IBS symptoms, see your health care provider. A fever higher than 100.5°F, along with IBS symptoms, needs professional evaluation. Weight loss is not a symptom of IBS. Sometimes, people believe their diarrhea results in weight loss. Small weight changes are common for most people. If you begin to steadily lose weight without trying, that is a signal to see your health care provider.

How Is IBS Treated?

The symptoms of IBS can affect many different areas of your life. Treating IBS focuses on getting your symptoms under control.

Drug Treatment

There is no known drug treatment that will cure IBS. However, some medications are used to treat specific symptoms such as gas, constipation, and diarrhea. We explain what these medications do and how they are used in the Appendix.

The medicines can help you feel better, but none of them will make your IBS go away.

Symptom Management

Self-management strategies have been tested in studies and found to be useful for symptom control in IBS. These techniques are easy to learn, and with a little practice, you can make them part of your daily routine. This book will help you learn symptom self-management strategies in three different areas: managing what you eat, building relaxation skills, and learning new ways of thinking. These strategies will give you a foundation for managing your IBS symptoms.

Stress and IBS

What Is Stress?

In 1946, a researcher named Hans Seyle coined the word *stress* to mean "the nonspecific response of the body to any demand placed on it." Today, we typically use the word stress when describing the unpleasant feelings of physical tension, pressure, anxiety, or fatigue that occur when demands placed on us exceed our ability to cope. The demands that cause us to feel stressed are called *stressors*. Anything that we experience that demands a change, adjustment, or response from us is a stressor. The stress response is a physical and psychological reaction to stressors.

The Stress Response

The stress response prepares people to deal with real dangers. At one time, these dangers may have been unfriendly neighbors or life-threatening animals. When we perceive a threat, our bodies react swiftly to allow us to protect ourselves by either fighting or running away. We call this the *fight-or-flight* response or the *stress* response.

In the modern world, people only rarely experience life-threatening danger. Most of us experience threats in more subtle ways. If you are at risk of losing your job, had an angry conversation with your spouse, or have just run out of gas on the highway, your frustration or anxiety may activate the stress response. Our bodies protect us and can't distinguish between an angry bear and an angry boss. We are built to react to either threat in the same way.

When you interpret a situation as dangerous, the stress response is activated. A cascade of changes takes place within your body. Cortisol and adrenaline are released into the bloodstream; they provide you with extra energy. Blood pressure and heart rate increase, supplying blood to large muscle groups and increasing muscle tension. Breathing speeds up, increasing the oxygen supply. The blood supply is diverted away from the digestive, immune, and reproductive systems, giving more blood to the large muscles, heart, and lungs that are necessary to fight or flee. All of these changes happen automatically or involuntarily.

The Stress Response and IBS

Studies have shown that there is a connection between your brain and your intestines. This is called the *brain-gut* connection. When your brain interprets a situation as a threat, it can lead to changes in the intestines. Exaggerated bowel contractions may cause cramping, bloating, or diarrhea. If the forward motion of the bowels decreases, stools can become hard and difficult to pass, leading to constipation.

Most stressors come and go. The human body is built to spring back and return to normal when the stressor is gone. When stress is chronic, repeated, and severe, the disruption can be greater. During long-term stress, the intestines are given repeated messages to speed up or slow down. After a while, the mechanisms for regulating normal functioning are affected. The digestive tract becomes overly sensitive, reacting to low levels of stimulation with strong reactions.

Fortunately, we can use our minds to distinguish what our instincts cannot. Although the stress response is involuntary, everyone is able to take some control over it. We want you to learn how to interpret situations as manageable problems rather than threats. By increasing the awareness of what your body is doing, you can slow your breathing and relax your muscles. This allows you to quiet the stress response.

In other words, you can take control of how you interpret a situation and choose to react to it. By taking control, you can approach stressful situations more calmly. This allows your body to relax and provides a way to decrease your IBS symptoms.

Triggers

There are many things that cause or "trigger" symptoms and influence communication between the brain and gut. There are physical stressors such as heat, cold, spicy foods, fatigue, or hunger that test our bodies. Emotional stressors such as ending a relationship, a heavy workload, holiday preparations, or an argument with a friend can leave us feeling overwhelmed or distressed. Losing a job or the death of a spouse are major stressors that can have a significant impact on anyone. Environmental stressors such as a noisy or polluted workplace, flashing lights, or rush-hour traffic can leave us overstimulated and agitated.

It's interesting that what feels stressful to one person may not bother someone else. Think about a 12-year-old thoroughly enjoying a video arcade, while his parents stand by wishing for earplugs and experiencing headaches. Likewise, some people enjoy a traffic jam because it means they have a few extra minutes to listen to music and relax before getting home to make dinner. It is not the situation itself that is stressful; it is your reaction to it.

All people have certain triggers that cause them to get anxious, angry, or depressed. If you can learn to react differently to these triggers, you can control your stress level and reduce your IBS symptoms.

Learning Relaxation Skills

Relaxation is the opposite of stress. You can't be relaxed and stressed at the same time. When you relax, you reverse the effects of the stress response. Your blood pressure comes down, your heart rate returns to normal, your breathing is slower and deeper, muscle tension lessens, and blood returns to the stomach and intestines.

Learning to relax is one way you can manage your response to stress. There are many ways to relax. You can even learn to relax in a stressful situation. Relaxation consists of calming your mind and body. Decreasing muscle tension, slowing your breathing, and changing your thoughts to healthy, productive ways of thinking are all a part of learning to relax and reverse the stress response.

Relaxation is a natural state that your body can instinctively attain. It is only chronic stress and lack of skills that keep you from being able to relax. You can learn and practice activities and skills to help you relax.

Any activity that results in a release of tension or calms the body can be helpful in relaxation. For some people, activities such as walking or swimming can release tension. Calming hobbies such as sewing, woodworking, gardening, and yoga; prayer or meditation; listening to quiet music; or relaxation exercises help to calm the mind and body.

If you have lived with chronic stress, learning to relax takes time and practice, but you can master it. Learning to keep your mind and body calm through relaxation is one of the most important ways of decreasing your IBS symptoms. We have seen the difference that doing this can make! After working through the 8 weeks of our treatment program, more than half of study participants had fewer days with moderate to severe pain or discomfort. About 40% had fewer days with additional symptoms, such as bloating, diarrhea, constipation, urgency, or intestinal gas. These positive changes lasted for as long as we followed participants after the treatment ended, as long as 9 months. So, we are convinced that this can work for you, too.

Abdominal Breathing Exercise

- Begin by lying on your back in a quiet place, wearing loose clothes. In this position, you may do abdominal breathing naturally. You may feel more comfortable with your knees bent or with a pillow under your knees.
- Place one hand lightly on your chest and the other hand lightly on your abdomen below your belt line.
- Exhale.
- Inhale slowly to the count of 3 or 4, feeling your abdomen rise. Your chest should be still.
- Exhale slowly to the count of 5 or 6, using your abdominal muscles and diaphragm. When you exhale, you should feel your abdomen fall.

Abdominal Breathing

Abdominal breathing is a type of slow, deep breathing that uses your abdominal muscles and diaphragm. Most people breathe with their shoulder and chest muscles. Take a deep breath. Do your shoulders go up? Does your chest rise? This type of chest breathing leads to rapid, shallow breathing. Chest breathing is such an ingrained habit for most people that it may take a few days of practice to feel comfortable with abdominal breathing. The reward will be great, though, when you learn to relax.

Begin your abdominal breathing by exhaling, which will make it easier to take a slow deep abdominal breath. It is sometimes helpful to imagine that your abdomen is like a balloon. When you inhale, the balloon inflates and your abdomen rises. When you exhale, the balloon deflates and your abdomen falls.

Practice this type of breathing at a slow, relaxed pace, exhaling slower than you inhale. For example, you may inhale to the count of 4 and exhale to the count of 6. Choose numbers that are comfortable for you and gradually try to make the exhale even longer.

When you master this type of breathing, try it in a sitting and standing position. Then begin looking for opportunities during your day to do the breathing. Try using it every time you are waiting, when you are on hold on the telephone, when the computer is warming up, when you are in line in the grocery store, and when you are waiting for the kids to get in the car. As you increase the number of times during the day that you practice abdominal breathing, you will begin to feel more relaxed and gain increased control over your IBS symptoms.

The Quieting Response

The quieting response was developed by Charles Stroebel in the 1980s to help people manage stress. Our version of the quieting response is a mini-relaxation exercise that you can use anytime and anywhere that you feel stress coming on. It only requires you to have mastered abdominal breathing. You can do this exercise either standing or sitting.

Once you learn abdominal breathing and the quieting response, you will find that they are skills that you can use throughout your day. You can do either or both of these when you are standing, sitting, talking on the phone, before meals, or even during a stressful conversation with your boss. Although it can be very pleasant and sometimes useful to find a quiet spot to recline and do these exercises, one important benefit is that they can be done throughout your day and they can be done during each crisis that you face. Study participants who had suffered from IBS for years were surprised at what such simple exercises did to help them manage their symptoms.

> ## Quieting Response Exercise
>
> Take one slow, deep abdominal breath. As you exhale, let your mind relax. Say to yourself, any of the following:
>
> "Alert mind, calm body."
> "I'm going to keep my body out of this."
> "Quiet mind, quiet body."
> "Relax."
>
> Take a second slow, deep abdominal breath. As you exhale, let your jaw and shoulders drop and feel a wave of warmth flowing through your body.

Skill Building

The goal of the next 8 weeks is for you to develop new skills that will help you manage your IBS symptoms. Skill building involves learning and practicing new skills, strategies, and techniques in dietary management, relaxation skills, and healthy thought patterns.

There are two steps in this process. The first step focuses on self-awareness. We want you to keep track of your IBS symptoms so you can begin to identify patterns and factors that make them better or worse. For this, you will use the Keeping Track forms. You can fill in the Keeping Track forms at the back of the book for this, or you can make copies.

We want you to make time to complete this form each evening, so you can reflect on the day and score your symptoms. The information you put on the form will help you identify the relationship between your symptoms and factors such as diet, stress, and thought patterns. You will also use this form as you learn stress management skills, so you can track the changes in your symptoms. We will explain how to review and interpret the information you collect with this form on a regular basis so you can identify the patterns.

The Keeping Track forms will help you to monitor your symptoms. It is difficult for people to recall what their symptoms were like two weeks ago. When study participants completed the 8 weeks of keeping track, they were often surprised at the changes in their symptoms!

Not all of the strategies will effectively reduce symptoms for everyone. By keeping track and completing a form every evening on which you rank your symptoms on the corresponding days, it becomes easy to identify which strategies are the most effective for you.

Rebecca tried to practice and complete all of the "homework" throughout the 8 weeks she participated in the study. But life had a way of interfering. She would get busy, forget, or (at the beginning) wasn't even sure how she was supposed to practice or when or where. Again, "playing detective" with why things were not progressing as fast as she would like, she learned to be more specific with her homework, tried to set up reminders, and paced herself better. When we reviewed her Keeping Track forms at the end of the 8 weeks, she was surprised to see that her abdominal pain and constipation, which had ranged from moderate to severe in the first few weeks of the study, were now absent or mild on most days. She did not remember how severe the symptoms had been! She was aware, however, that her IBS symptoms were no longer the center of her life by the end of the study. Her Keeping Track forms were a great reminder of the progress she had made.

The second step in building your IBS management skills is developing a plan of action:

Action Plan

What will I do?

When will I do it?

What obstacles might prevent me from reaching my goal?

How will I avoid these obstacles?

Our patient Anil decided that his goal was to practice the quieting response this week. He wanted to do it 4 times each day, before breakfast, lunch, and dinner and at bedtime. However, Anil was concerned that he might forget. His solution was to set the alarm on his cell phone to ring at these times. Anil used the Keeping Track form daily to record his symptoms and his quieting response practice. Take a look at Anil's Keeping Track form after a week (page 18).

You will have specific tasks to complete each week. These tasks help you learn and practice new skills for managing your symptoms. The tasks are broken into steps that are manageable and easy to learn. It's important that you track your symptoms, responses, and results on the Keeping Track forms.

When you complete the program, you will have a long-term plan using skills that you have found effective in managing your symptoms.

How to Keep Track

We know from past studies that people are not very good at remembering how their symptoms change over time. You may have never bothered to track them before. To support your tracking efforts, there are blank Keeping Track forms for you in the back of this book. This will take about 5 minutes to complete each day.

On this form, you will rate your average level of abdominal pain, diarrhea, constipation, bloating, and stress as none, 0; mild, 1; moderate 2; and severe 3. You will also record the strategies that you are using. For example, you may be assigned to do the quieting response 3 times a day. In the left column you will write "QR 3×/day." Under the day of the week you will write the number of times you actually did the quieting response. Over a period of time, you will be able to track the effectiveness of the strategies you are learning and determine which ones are most effective.

Anil's Keeping Track Form, Week 1

Circle the average level of discomfort you experienced for each symptom over the past 24 hours: 0, none; 1, mild; 2, moderate; 3, severe. Use the left column to write your goals for this week.

DATE	Feb. 2	Feb. 3	Feb. 4	Feb. 5	Feb. 6	Feb. 7	Feb. 8
Abdominal pain	3 2 ①　0	3 ②　1 0	③ 2 1 0	3 ②　1 0	3 ②　1 0	③ 2 1 0	3 ②　1 0
Diarrhea	3 2 ①　0	3 2 ①　0	3 ②　1 0	③ 2 1 0	3 ②　1 0	3 ②　1 0	3 ②　1 0
Constipation	3 2 1 ⓪	3 2 ①　0	3 2 1 ⓪	3 2 1 ⓪	3 2 1 ⓪	3 2 1 ⓪	3 ②　1 0
Bloating	3 2 ①　0	3 ②　1 0	3 ②　1 0	3 2 ①　0	3 2 ①　0	3 ②　1 0	3 ②　1 0
Stress	3 2 ①　0	3 ②　1 0	3 ②　1 0	3 ②　1 0	3 ②　1 0	③ 2 1 0	3 ②　1 0

My goals this week:

	Feb. 2	Feb. 3	Feb. 4	Feb. 5	Feb. 6	Feb. 7	Feb. 8
Abdominal breathing 2 minutes each morning and evening	(Yes) No #*2*	(Yes) No #*2*	(Yes) No #*1*	(Yes) No #*2*	(Yes) No #*2*	Yes No #*2*	(Yes) No #*2*
Quieting response 2 to 3 times each day	Yes (No) #___	(Yes) No #*2*	(Yes) No #*3*	(Yes) No #*3*	(Yes) No #*2*	(Yes) No #*2*	(Yes) No #*2*
	Yes No #___	Yes No #___	Yes No #___	Yes No #___	Yes No #___	Yes No #___	Yes No #___
	Yes No #___	Yes No #___	Yes No #___	Yes No #___	Yes No #___	Yes No #___	Yes No #___

Keeping Track Form

Circle the average level of discomfort you experienced for each symptom over the past 24 hours: 0, none; 1, mild; 2, moderate; 3, severe. Use the left column to write your goals for this week.

DATE							
Abdominal pain	3 2 1 0	3 2 1 0	3 2 1 0	3 2 1 0	3 2 1 0	3 2 1 0	3 2 1 0
Diarrhea	3 2 1 0	3 2 1 0	3 2 1 0	3 2 1 0	3 2 1 0	3 2 1 0	3 2 1 0
Constipation	3 2 1 0	3 2 1 0	3 2 1 0	3 2 1 0	3 2 1 0	3 2 1 0	3 2 1 0
Bloating	3 2 1 0	3 2 1 0	3 2 1 0	3 2 1 0	3 2 1 0	3 2 1 0	3 2 1 0
Stress	3 2 1 0	3 2 1 0	3 2 1 0	3 2 1 0	3 2 1 0	3 2 1 0	3 2 1 0
My goals this week:							
	Yes No #___	Yes No #___	Yes No #___	Yes No #___	Yes No #___	Yes No #___	Yes No #___
	Yes No #___	Yes No #___	Yes No #___	Yes No #___	Yes No #___	Yes No #___	Yes No #___
	Yes No #___	Yes No #___	Yes No #___	Yes No #___	Yes No #___	Yes No #___	Yes No #___
	Yes No #___	Yes No #___	Yes No #___	Yes No #___	Yes No #___	Yes No #___	Yes No #___

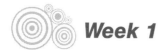 ## *Week 1*

Skills to Build

Relaxation

Practice abdominal breathing for 2 minutes in the morning before you get up and for 2 minutes in the evening after you go to bed.

Practice the quieting response 2 to 3 times a day.

Self-Awareness

Complete the Keeping Track form each day.

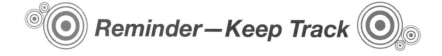

Reminder—Keep Track

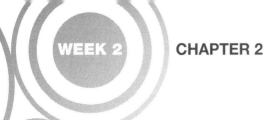

A New Approach to Your Food

IN THIS CHAPTER

Learn about a healthy diet, including serving sizes and vitamin supplementation. Begin to keep a Food Journal.

QUICK FACTS

Eating a healthy, well-balanced diet is important in managing your IBS symptoms and in your overall health. A healthy diet emphasizes fruits, vegetables, whole grains, low-fat or fat-free dairy products, lean proteins, and a small amount of healthy oils.

It is common for people with IBS to restrict their diet as a way of managing their symptoms.

A healthy diet and lifestyle include regular physical activity, moderation, personalization, portion size, variety, and gradual improvement.

Most people find that their IBS symptoms decrease if they eat small, frequent meals beginning with breakfast. To eat every 3 to 4 hours, you need to plan ways to work snacks into your day.

Food and Your IBS

What you eat, when you eat, how you eat, and how you feel are related, in part, to your symptoms of IBS. The exact nature of this relationship differs among individuals. Your symptoms may be tightly connected to how and what you eat. Maybe you already avoid ice cream, coffee, or popcorn because you always get unpleasant results. Yet someone else is unable to detect any pattern among foods, eating patterns, and symptoms. So, we cannot recommend one single diet for all people with IBS.

You can investigate suspected diet-related IBS symptoms in four easy steps. Completing these steps will help you understand and manage your symptoms.

1. Begin eating a healthy, balanced diet.
2. Eat small, frequent meals.
3. Identify foods and eating habits that trigger symptoms.
4. Decide which changes in your diet will be the most beneficial for you.

What Is Healthy Eating?

Research shows that the human body requires specific nutrients in specific amounts to feel well, function at its best, and cope with stress. If the way you eat supplies these nutrients in the correct amounts, you are eating healthy. You are balancing your body's needs with the fuel you supply. Are you functioning at your best?

Most of us can use some improvement in the healthy eating arena. But don't start a rigid diet or deny yourself all of your favorite foods. You need to come up with a plan that you can and want to follow most of the time. The key to a healthy diet is eating foods that are nutrient rich.

Eat a variety of nutritious foods in balanced amounts and don't eat too much or too little of one food group. We will explain which foods are nutrient rich and what a healthy amount is.

Tips for Healthy Eating with IBS

Don't skip meals, especially breakfast, and eat smaller, more frequent meals. Many participants in our study found that eating large and/or high-calorie meals affected bowel motility, which brought on cramping or diarrhea. Many found that they avoided IBS symptoms if they ate every 3 to 4 hours while awake. This means including a small breakfast in your day, eating less at each meal, and adding small snacks midmorning, midafternoon, and before bedtime. This way, you are not increasing your calories—you are spreading them more evenly throughout the day. If you begin to keep healthy snacks in your car, briefcase, purse, desk, and refrigerator, this will be much easier. You will probably find it helpful to make a written plan of how you will go about this before you start. Expect to encounter a few obstacles that will interfere with your plan.

Take the time to eat and chew slowly. When you eat quickly, you may not fully chew the food, and gulping it down makes you swallow extra air. This makes it harder for the stomach to break down the food, and the extra air causes a bloating feeling. Eating too fast or eating on the run can cause indigestion. Indigestion is stomachache, bloating, reflux, and heartburn.

Take a few relaxed deep breaths before eating. IBS symptoms are generally worse when people feel stressed. Breathing deeply for a short time before you eat calms the body and improves digestion.

Choose a place to eat that is relaxing. At work, try to eat away from your desk. At home, once you have prepared a meal, sit down and relax while you eat. Positive, pleasant conversation over dinner is helpful in making mealtimes relaxing, so turn off the TV. This is not the time to talk about your problems at work or to discipline the children. When everyone is finished with the meal, relax for a few minutes before moving to your next activity.

Keep healthy snacks available throughout the day. You can keep a "portable" snack in your purse, briefcase, desk at work, car, locker at school, refrigerator, or even in your pocket. Having a healthy snack between meals, mid-morning, and afternoon will help you to eat every 3 to 4 hours. Try a variety of snacks to keep them interesting.

Limit alcohol. Beer, wine, and other alcoholic drinks trigger IBS symptoms in some people. If you drink alcohol, we recommend limiting your intake to one drink per day with a meal. Alcohol can promote diarrhea.

Avoid sorbitol. Sorbitol is a sweetener used in many low-sugar diet foods, especially candy, gum, breath mints, and some prepared foods. It is hard for some people to digest, causing abdominal pain, bloating, and/or diarrhea.

Healthy Snack Ideas

- applesauce and other fruit in individual containers
- cereal with low-fat milk, rice milk, or soy milk
- baked or low-fat crackers
- low-fat yogurt
- fresh fruit that you can tolerate
- small amounts (¼ cup) of dried fruit that you can tolerate
- pretzels
- rice cakes
- digestive baby cookies
- low-fat fruit-filled cookies
- whole-wheat toast
- small bagel with low-fat cream cheese or a small amount of jam
- baked potato
- rice
- ready-to-eat carrots

Table 1. Caffeine in Food and Beverages

Beverage (12 oz.) or Food	Amount of Caffeine
coffee	220–360 mg
tea	80 mg
Jolt	70 mg
Mountain Dew	55 mg
Coke, Diet Coke	45 mg
Pepsi, Diet Pepsi	37 mg
chocolate in candy, desserts, and beverages	5–10 mg/serving

Limit coffee and caffeine. Coffee, with or without caffeine, can cause diarrhea and can make IBS symptoms worse. If coffee aggravates your IBS symptoms, try cutting down on the amount you drink each day and avoid drinking it first thing in the morning or on an empty stomach. Also, consider cutting down on the amount of caffeine you drink or switching to decaffeinated beverages (Table 1).

An Easy, Personalized Healthy Eating Plan

MyPyramid, Steps to a Healthier You (www.MyPyramid.gov) is a tool from the U.S. Department of Agriculture (USDA) that helps you choose a diet that's right for you. MyPyramid is based on USDA research on what foods Americans typically eat, the nutrients in these foods, and how to make the best food choices. All types of foods are included on the pyramid, even foods that should be eaten sparingly such as fats and sugar. Surveys of the average American diet indicate that most people eat too many fatty foods and not enough fruits and vegetables.

A healthy diet emphasizes nutrient-rich foods: fruits, vegetables, whole grains, and fat-free or low-fat dairy products. A healthy diet also includes lean meats (lean cuts of beef are round, chuck, loin, and sirloin; lean pork cuts are tenderloin or loin chops), poultry, fish, cooked dried beans, eggs, and nuts (if tolerated). Use foods high in saturated fats and cholesterol, salt, and added sugar sparingly. Although a healthy diet is generally the best way to meet nutritional needs, adding a multivitamin or mineral or calcium supplement to your diet may also be a helpful way to meet vitamin and mineral requirements.

Each of the MyPyramid food groups provides some of the nutrients you need daily. But the actual amount of food you need daily varies depending on your age, sex, weight, height, and amount of daily physical activity. You can create a personalized healthy eating plan at www.MyPyramid.gov. Click on "My Pyramid Plan" and answer a few simple questions. You will receive a dietary plan that is personalized to you and your lifestyle.

Alexandra skipped breakfast and didn't eat until early afternoon each day. She did this because she knew that her IBS symptoms would start after her first meal. The longer she waited to eat, the longer she could put off the pain and diarrhea.

It was not easy for her to try eating small, frequent meals because it seemed to Alexandra like she would be letting go of the only control she had over her symptoms. But she agreed to give it a try. Alexandra began eating a half a piece of toast each morning after she got up. At about 10:00 a.m., she ate a half a banana. Alexandra was surprised that she wasn't very hungry at lunch time, but she ate part of her sandwich and the rest of her banana for lunch. At 3:00 p.m., she had a carton of yogurt and a few crackers. By the time she picked up her kids from after school activities and got dinner on the table, it was often 7:00 p.m. In the past, her IBS symptoms were often at their peak by dinner. With her new eating routine, she was feeling better. At dinner, she ate about half of the portion she generally had, then she ate a handful of pretzels before she went to bed. Of course, each day did not go perfectly. Sometimes her schedule, or her children, seemed to pressure her into following an old pattern. This was easier, because it was so familiar. But over time she came to see that the old pattern also produced the old symptom pattern! She asked for support from those around her to keep the new system in place.

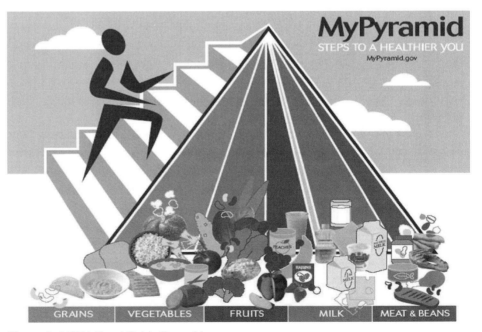

Figure 1. USDA Food Guide Pyramid

Over the next several weeks, when she followed her new system more consistently, Alexandra was surprised that her midafternoon abdominal pain began to decrease significantly. This eating pattern gave her a new sense of control over her IBS symptoms. Now she keeps snacks in her purse, glove compartment, and desk drawer so it's easier for her to eat on a regular basis.

Nutritional Value of Foods

For good health, you need foods from each food group (Figure 1). Despite what many fad diets suggest, it is not healthy to eliminate certain food groups and overeat from another group.

Bread, cereals, rice, and pasta group. This group provides complex carbohydrates that fuel the body. They are rich in iron and B vitamins, especially thiamin, riboflavin, niacin, and folate. Whole grains, such as whole wheat bread, oatmeal, brown rice, and whole-grain pastas, supply fiber. Grains are generally tolerated by people with IBS unless they have gluten intolerance or celiac disease. If you feel that you are sensitive to gluten, it is important to see your health care provider for an assessment. Untreated celiac disease damages the small intestine.

Vegetable group. This group provides a variety of nutrients, including carbohydrates, vitamins A and C, fiber, and minerals such as potassium. Cooked dried beans, such as navy, lima, and kidney beans, are considered vegetables, although they supply protein and are also included in the meat group. People with IBS can usually tolerate many different vegetables such as squash, peas, spinach, carrots, green beans, beets, cucumber, and sweet potato.

Fruit group. Fruits and fruit juices provide vitamins A and C, minerals, fiber, and potassium. Canned fruits, ripe bananas, peaches, plums, grapes, blueberries, and applesauce are all fruits that are widely available and easily tolerated by those with IBS. Only 100% fruit juice counts as fruit. Most fruit drinks contain very little fruit juice and lots of added sugar.

Milk, cheese, and yogurt group. Milk products are very nutritious, providing calcium, protein, riboflavin, phosphorus, and vitamins A and D. Often, individuals with IBS can tolerate low-fat or fat-free milk products.

Both cheese and yogurt contain substantially less milk sugar (lactose) per serving than a serving of liquid milk. Yogurt with live and active cultures is the healthiest yogurt; look for the National Yogurt Association's live and active culture

(LAC) seal. The live cultures are bacteria that change milk into yogurt. These bacteria can improve digestion because they help promote a balance of microorganisms in the gastrointestinal tract. Many brands, including Dannon, Nancy's, and Yoplait, carry the LAC seal.

Suggestions for Low-Fat Dairy

Fat-free milk

1% milk

Fat-free or low-fat yogurt

Fat-free or low-fat cheese

Fat-free cottage cheese

Fat-free or light sour cream

Meat, poultry, dried beans, eggs, and nuts group. The foods in this group supply protein, B vitamins, iron, and zinc. Meats can be high in fat. To lower fat content, choose lean cuts of meat such as "USDA Select" beef round, sirloin, flank steak, and tenderloin; chicken or turkey without the skin (or remove the skin after cooking and before eating); pork tenderloin; or fish.

If you are a vegetarian, avoiding beans and nuts lowers your protein intake. It is possible to eat a healthy, well-balanced diet and manage your IBS symptoms effectively by using the Vegetarian Diet Pyramid (www.oldwayspt. org/vegetarian_pyramid.html). You may find it helpful to consult a dietitian or nutritionist to provide additional information on healthy alternatives.

Fats, oils, and sweets group. These foods are a normal part of our diet, and the oils are important for supplying the omega fatty acids that healthy bodies need. It's healthier to eat solid fats and sugars sparingly. To reduce solid fats and sugars, choose lower-fat foods from the first five food groups and use small amounts of sugar and fats when you cook. Be aware of how much fat (such as butter) and sugar (including honey and syrup) you add to foods at the table. Most people with IBS feel better on a low-fat diet. Limit how often you choose to eat high-sugar foods such as sweet desserts, candy, or regular soft drinks. Many people also find that they feel better when they decrease the amount of sugar in their diet.

What Is a Serving?

Your personalized MyPyramid gives you the number of daily servings to choose from each food group based on the amount of daily calories you need. Table 2 provides serving sizes per day based on a typical 2,000-calorie diet. The number of servings will vary with calorie requirements, but the serving sizes always remain consistent.

Table 2. Daily Servings of Food Groups

Food Groups	USDA Food Guide Amount	Equivalent Amounts
Fruit	2 cups (4 servings)	A ½-cup equivalent is: • ½ cup fresh, frozen, or canned fruit • 1 medium fruit • ¼ cup dried fruit • ½ cup vegetable juice
Vegetable • Dark green vegetable • Orange vegetable • Legumes • Starchy vegetable • Additional vegetables	2.5 cups (5 servings) • 3 cups/week • 2 cups/week • 3 cups/week • 3 cups/week • 6.5 cups/week	A ½-cup equivalent is: • ½ cup cut up, raw or cooked • 1 cup raw leafy • ½ cup vegetable juice
Grain • Whole grains • Other grains	6 1-oz. equivalents • 3 1-oz. equivalents • 3 1-oz. equivalents	A 1-oz. equivalent is: • 1 slice bread • 1 cup dry cereal • ½ cup cooked rice, pasta, cereal, or grain
Meat and Beans	5.5 1-oz. equivalents	A 1-oz. equivalent is: • 1 oz. of cooked lean meat, poultry, or fish • 1 egg • ¼ cup cooked dried beans or tofu • 1 Tbsp. peanut butter • ½ oz. nuts or seeds
Milk	3 cups	A 1-cup equivalent is: • 1 cup fat-free/low-fat milk, yogurt • 1½ oz. fat-free, low-fat, or reduced fat natural cheese • 2 oz. fat-free/low-fat processed cheese
Oils	27 grams (6 tsp.)	Most Americans consume enough oil in the foods they eat such as nuts, fish, cooking oil, and salad dressing. • 1 Tbsp. low-fat mayo • 2 Tbsp. light salad dressing • 1 tsp. vegetable oil
Discretionary Calorie Allowance	276 calories	

Estimating serving sizes (Table 3) can be challenging, and many foods are packaged in sizes much larger than we realize. For example, a large bagel or muffin can be 4 or 5 ounces, which is equivalent to 4 or 5 bread and cereal servings. Table 3 lists some guides to help you estimate size of servings.

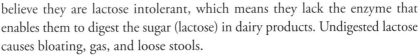

Table 3. Estimating Serving Sizes

Size	Serving Size Equivalent
1 thumb or 4 stacked dice	1 oz. cheese
Small matchbook	1 oz. meat (cooked)
1 deck of cards or bar of soap	3 oz. meat (cooked)
Palm of hand	3 oz. meat (cooked)
1 ice cream scoop	½ cup
Fist	1 cup
Handful	1–2 oz. of a snack food
Tennis ball	1 medium fruit serving
Computer mouse	1 medium potato
Ping pong ball	2 Tbsp. peanut butter

Which Vitamins and Minerals Might You Lack?

Lots of people in the United States don't get enough dietary calcium in general, and many people with IBS avoid dairy products. Often, they believe they are lactose intolerant, which means they lack the enzyme that enables them to digest the sugar (lactose) in dairy products. Undigested lactose causes bloating, gas, and loose stools.

IBS and lactose intolerance are two different health issues. You may have IBS and you may have lactose intolerance—but you don't have lactose intolerance because you have IBS. Often, people with IBS find that the fat in dairy products triggers their symptoms. This is an important difference because most people with IBS can tolerate fat-free or low-fat dairy products. If you are able to tolerate these foods, it's much easier to get the recommended number of servings of dairy into your diet each day.

If you are concerned, however, that you may be lactose intolerant, it is important to discuss this with your health care provider and get tested if appropriate. You can also try an elimination diet on your own (see Sidebar).

You, like many people with IBS, might avoid dairy or be on a restricted diet that limits dairy foods. For example, Debra avoids most dairy products but occasionally has a latte with fat-free milk. Sundara eats yogurt several times a week but avoids most other dairy products. If you are limiting your dairy intake, you are likely not getting enough calcium (Table 4) or vitamin D.

Table 4. Daily Calcium Requirements

19 to 50 years old	1,000 mg/day
51 and older	1,200 mg/day

Elimination Diet for Lactose Intolerance

Perhaps you experience excessive diarrhea, gas, or bloating after eating dairy products and are concerned that you may be lactose intolerant. You may first want to try switching to only fat-free or 1% dairy products. If this does not relieve or significantly reduce your symptoms, consider trying an elimination diet or visiting your doctor for further testing.

As the name suggests, you would eliminate all dairy products from your diet for 1 to 2 weeks. Foods to avoid are milk, yogurt, cheese, ice cream, cottage cheese, or sour cream. You may use soymilk or rice milk as a milk substitute, and butter is safe to use. After a continuous period with no dairy products, drink a large glass (12–16 ounces) of fat-free milk. If you experience a lot of gas, bloating, or diarrhea within an hour or two after drinking the milk, discuss your results with your primary health care provider or dietitian. They may suggest that you undergo formal testing for lactose intolerance. You might instead decide to avoid dairy products on a regular basis.

You can substitute lactose-free products such as Lactaid for dairy. Many people with lactose intolerance switch to soy and rice milk products. These are clearly labeled in your grocery store. You may be able to tolerate these lactose-free dairy products or use a lactase enzyme supplement, a tablet that helps your system digest the lactose in milk. If you go dairy free, you will need to pay attention to your calcium intake and probably add a supplement.

These nutrients don't directly influence your IBS symptoms, but maintaining a healthy lifestyle requires eating a balanced diet that includes these nutrients. The recommended amount of calcium depends on your age. If you don't get enough dairy, you can add a calcium and vitamin D supplement to your diet.

Foods that are high in calcium include milk, yogurt, tofu, collard and turnip greens, broccoli, bok choy, kale, pinto beans, figs, and canned salmon and sardines with bones. Calcium-fortified orange juice and breakfast cereals are also good sources of calcium. You can estimate your calcium intake by using the "rule of 300s." Give yourself 300 mg of calcium for a well-balanced diet and add 300 mg for each cup of milk or yogurt or 1.5 oz cheese or 4 oz of tofu. Thus, someone who eats a balanced diet that includes a carton of yogurt and 8 ounces of milk each day consumes approximately 900 mg of calcium.

If you do not eat dairy products or regularly consume calcium-fortified foods, consider taking a calcium supplement. Note that your body can absorb only 500–600 mg of calcium at a time, so if you take more, split the doses with several hours in between. We recommend that you look for a product that includes calcium citrate (a chelated form that is easy to absorb) or calcium carbonate (a form that requires adequate stomach acid for digestion).

Proper absorption of calcium requires magnesium and vitamin D, so consider a multivitamin supplement that contains both of these. Note that iron competes with calcium for absorption, so find a multivitamin without iron and avoid taking a calcium supplement soon after eating meat. The other fact to note about calcium is that it can bulk up the stool. For those troubled by loose stools, this is helpful. But for those troubled by constipation, using a calcium supplement that also contains magnesium is helpful in another way: magnesium tends to have a laxative effect, which counteracts the constipating nature of calcium supplements.

Many people are deficient in vitamin D and don't realize it. More doctors are routinely measuring blood levels of vitamin D in their patients. Research suggests that vitamin D helps provide protection from osteoporosis, high blood pressure, heart disease, several types of cancer, and autoimmune diseases. Those most at risk for vitamin D deficiency are elderly, dark-skinned, or obese individuals; exclusively breast-fed infants; and those who cover all exposed skin or use sunscreen whenever outside. As little as 10 minutes of daily exposure to sunlight is enough to prevent vitamin D deficiency. Your doctor can check your blood level and determine if you need a vitamin D supplement. Food sources of vitamin D are fatty fish (salmon, mackerel, tuna), eggs, fortified milk, cod liver oil, and breakfast cereals fortified with vitamin D. The typical American diet supplies about 100 international units (IUs) of vitamin D each day. Recent research indicates that this is likely inadequate.

A well-balanced diet is part of a healthy lifestyle and helps effectively manage IBS symptoms. A multivitamin or a multivitamin with minerals can also be helpful. Choose a vitamin that meets the standards of the United States Pharmacopeia (shown with USP on the label). If you choose a multivitamin with minerals, it should contain both copper and zinc (not just one) and the iron amount should not exceed 18 mg for women and 10 mg for men. Health care providers often recommend iron for menstruating women. Look for supplements with close to 100% Daily Value level for the vitamins.

Avoid high-potency supplements and those that require taking several pills each day. It is best to take vitamins with, or immediately after, meals to enhance absorption (with the exception of mixing iron and calcium).

It costs approximately $50 to $75 a year to take a multivitamin every day. You can buy vitamins at the supermarket, drug store, health food store, or online. The best bargains

Sample Multivitamins

Centrum
Nature Made Essential Tablets Daily
One A Day Women's Tablets
One A Day
Rite Aid Whole Source
Safeway Select OmniSource
Walgreen's Ultra Choice

are typically from large retailers like Costco, K-Mart, or Bartell's. These are great choices but there are many others.

Special Advice for Vegetarians

Be sure to include adequate amounts of protein, iron, calcium, zinc, and vitamin B$_{12}$ in your diet. The USDA provides guidelines for a well-balanced vegetarian diet in the guide MyPyramid, Steps to a Healthier You, 10 Tips for Following a Vegetarian Diet (www.MyPyramid.gov).

- Choose a wide variety of foods to meet your nutritional needs. Fruits and vegetables of many different colors will provide a wide variety of nutrients.
- Protein is an essential part of any diet. Meet your needs with plant-based foods such as nuts, peas, soy products, beans, lentils, and rice.
- Including calcium-fortified orange juice and breakfast cereals, soy products, and dark green leafy vegetables in your diet will help you meet your calcium needs.
- Get adequate vitamin E by eating sunflower seeds, almonds, and hazelnuts as snacks or adding nuts to a salad or entreé on a regular basis.
- Vegetarian food products are often lower in saturated fats and contain no cholesterol.

Your Food Journal

We want you to begin keeping a Food Journal. The journal will help you determine if you are eating a balanced diet. By completing the Food Journal for several days, you will begin to discover areas of your diet that need to be changed. You may need to increase or decrease your intake of specific food groups. As you become more aware of what you are eating, you can begin to identify foods and eating habits that may contribute to your IBS symptoms. The Food Journal then becomes a way to track changes in your diet and symptom patterns, as well as recording your progress as you make changes toward a healthier diet.

After completing the Food Journal for several days, you can begin to identify trigger foods, evaluate eating patterns, and count the number of servings from each food group that you have each day. With this knowledge you can slowly make changes that will improve your diet and help you manage your IBS symptoms.

Use a new page each day. You can use the pages provided in the back of this book for this, but consider making copies first so you have a lot of blank forms to create your Food Journal.

1. In the left column, record the time that you experience IBS symptoms, stress, or the time that you eat.
2. Record your symptoms in the second column, along with a rating of the severity.
   We suggest you use the following codes:
   P abdominal pain or cramping
   D diarrhea
   C constipation
   B bloating
   1 mild
   2 moderate
   3 severe
   For example, D-2 would indicate moderately bothersome diarrhea.
3. In the third column, rate your level of stress, using 1 for mild, 2 for moderate, and 3 for severe. It is helpful to make a note of the type of stress being experienced. For example, 3/presentation would indicate that you experienced severe stress as you gave a presentation.
4. In the Food column, write down everything you eat or drink each day, for 5 to 7 days, noting the time you ate. Be as specific as possible and include serving size. This information will reveal eating patterns and possible trigger foods. It will allow you to count the number of servings of each food group that you consume each day and track your fiber intake.
5. The final column is where you keep track of your fiber intake throughout the day. During Week 4, you will use the Fiber Content list to calculate the fiber in each food item. For now, we want you to concentrate on eating small, healthy meals, not counting the fiber.
6. At the bottom of the page, check off the number of servings of fruit, vegetables, and grains. Do the same for the glasses (8 oz.) of water or other liquids you drink.

Jill's Food Journal can be your guide. Jill works full time as a receptionist. Her job has become increasingly stressful over the past few months. She seldom feels that she has the time to take a lunch break. In fact, she considers it a "good day" when she has time to run downstairs and get a sandwich.

Over the past few months, Jill's abdominal pain, constipation, and diarrhea have increased. She is aware that stress triggers her symptoms but the role of food is more confusing. Sometimes a food will aggravate her symptoms and other times the same food doesn't bother her at all. She decided to keep a Food Journal to see if she can identify any patterns or new insights.

At the end of a week, review your Food Journal. You are looking for patterns. For example, in Jill's Food Journal, we can see that she drinks black coffee on an empty stomach and experiences pain soon afterward. Is this the case on other days also? Does coffee always cause pain when she drinks it on an empty stomach? Does she ever drink coffee with food or later in the day and have fewer or different symptoms? Jill wants to determine if coffee is always a trigger for her symptoms. Many people find that they are able to tolerate coffee if they have their first cup later in the morning after they have had some food.

Jill eats three large meals with no snacks. Is this the case every day? Are there any days on which she eats small, frequent meals and has less pain?

Jill does not seem to drink any water on this day. She needs to look at the other days in her Food Journal to find out if this is always the case. It is important to include 48 to 64 oz. of fluid in your diet each day. Some of this can come from foods and beverages that contain water.

Jill seems to experience pain 1 to 2 hours after each meal. Is this the case on other days also? It will help you to answer the following questions as you look for patterns in your Food Journal.

- Are you eating small, frequent meals on a regular basis?
- Does your diet include enough servings from each food group?
- What time of day do your symptoms most often occur?
- When are your symptoms most severe?
- Are there any foods that are always or almost always followed by IBS symptoms?
- Do certain types of stress increase your sensitivity to any particular foods?
- Do some kinds of stress consistently lead to significant IBS symptoms?
- Are you getting enough fiber? If not, do your symptoms increase over the next few days? We will help you answer this question in Week 4.

Use the pages in the back of the book for your Food Journal, or make copies of the blank page.

Jill's Food Journal

Date: *Monday, February 20*

Time	Symptoms	Stress level	Food	Fiber
6:00 a.m.		0	Coffee, 8 oz., black	
7:00			Toast, 1 slice whole wheat	
			1 medium banana	
7:30	P–2	2		
	D–1			
12:00 p.m.		2	Sandwich: 2 slices whole wheat bread, 2 oz. turkey, 1 slice Swiss cheese, lettuce, 2 Tbsp. mayo	
			About 10 potato chips	
			2 chocolate chip cookies (2" diameter)	
			12 oz. Diet Pepsi	
2:00	P–2	2		
6:30	B–2	1	1 cup cooked spaghetti, ½ cup marinara, 1 Tbsp. parmesan cheese	
			Salad: 1 cup lettuce, ¼ tomato, ¼ cucumber, 2 Tbsp. low-fat ranch dressing	
			1 slice French bread (1" thick)	
			³⁄₄ cup vanilla ice cream	
7:45	P–2			
	D–2			

Fruit (☑ ☐ ☐ ☐) ☐ ☐ Vegetables (☑ ☑ ☑ ☐ ☐) ☐ ☐ ☐ Grains (☑ ☑ ☑ ☑ ☑ ☑) ☐ ☐ ☐ ☐
Dairy (☑ ☑ ☐) ☐ ☐ Meats and Beans ☑ ☐ ☐ ☐ ☐ ☐ 8 oz. of water ☐ ☐ ☐ ☐ ☐ ☐ ☐ ☐
Symptoms: P, abdominal pain or cramping; D, diarrhea; C, constipation; B, bloating.
Rate pain and stress: 1 = mild; 2 = moderate; 3 = severe.

Food Journal

Date: _____

Time	Symptoms	Stress level	Food	Fiber

Fruit (☐ ☐ ☐ ☐) ☐ ☐ Vegetables (☐ ☐ ☐ ☐ ☐) ☐ ☐ ☐ Grains (☐ ☐ ☐ ☐ ☐ ☐) ☐ ☐ ☐ ☐
Dairy (☐ ☐ ☐) ☐ ☐ Meats and Beans ☐ ☐ ☐ ☐ ☐ 8 oz. of water ☐ ☐ ☐ ☐ ☐ ☐ ☐ ☐
Symptoms: P, abdominal pain or cramping; D, diarrhea; C, constipation; B, bloating.
Rate pain and stress: 1 = mild; 2 = moderate; 3 = severe.

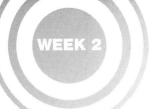
Trigger Foods

IN THIS CHAPTER

Learn how to identify foods that bring on your IBS symptoms.

QUICK FACTS

Trigger foods are foods that trigger IBS symptoms. By paying attention to and making notes about foods that you ate before your symptoms began with your Food Journal, you will be able to identify foods that trigger your symptoms.

Most people find that only a few foods trigger their symptoms and so only need to avoid those.

The most common foods that people with IBS avoid are high-fat dairy products, cruciferous vegetables (broccoli, cauliflower, Brussels sprouts, and cabbage), high-fat foods, spicy foods, beans, and coffee.

Do You Have a Trigger Food?

Trigger foods are foods that trigger symptoms. However, foods that act as triggers vary from person to person. Because so many factors influence IBS symptoms, it is difficult to determine which foods are problems. On a stressful day, you may have trouble tolerating pizza, but on your vacation it might not be a problem. For some women, certain foods may be a problem before their menstrual cycle. At other times of the month, these foods may be tolerated more easily. Just because a food has triggered symptoms once does not mean that particular food will always be a problem. In fact, as you learn to manage your symptoms using a variety of skills, the number of foods that you have difficulty tolerating may decrease.

An important part of your plan is to identify those foods that act as triggers for your IBS symptoms. There is a Trigger Foods list at the end of this chapter on which to make notes. The list may look long to you but it is important to realize that most people identify only a handful of foods that trigger their symptoms. There are foods that many people have told us, over and over again, are problems for them: high-fat dairy products, cruciferous vegetables (cabbage, broccoli, cauliflower, and Brussels sprouts), high-fat foods, beans, and coffee. Generally, people try to avoid the foods that cause their symptoms, but they seldom have to cut them out of their diet entirely. As IBS symptoms decrease, many people successfully add some of these foods back into their meals.

Krista has suffered with IBS for several years. The seemingly random pattern of her symptoms affected almost every area of her life. She had no idea when or why the severe diarrhea, intermittent constipation, and abdominal cramping would strike. To gain a sense of control over these symptoms, she began limiting her diet. She dreaded eating at all and only ate because it was a necessary part of life. Over time, she narrowed down the foods that she ate to chicken, rice, white bread, bananas, and applesauce. This diet helped to decrease her symptoms but it did not relieve them or give her a sense of control.

Identifying Trigger Foods

When you are able to identify the trigger foods that aggravate your IBS symptoms, you will probably begin to feel less concerned about your diet. Knowing which foods to avoid allows you to think differently about your diet and feel a greater sense of control. Although, you will probably only identify a handful of foods that bother you, there are a few food items in each food group that can be especially troublesome.

Dairy. Most people with IBS can tolerate low-fat dairy products. High-fat dairy products, such as whole milk, cheese made with whole milk, and regular ice cream, are often foods that people with IBS need to avoid or eat in small amounts.

Vegetables. The cruciferous vegetables—broccoli, cauliflower, cabbage, and Brussels sprouts—may cause gas, bloating, and abdominal pain. Some people tolerate cooked vegetables better than they tolerate fresh vegetables. Salads can occasionally be a problem for people with IBS. This is sometimes due to high-fat salad dressings.

Fruit. Unpeeled apples and pears can be a trigger food for some people. Citrus fruit is occasionally a trigger food for people with IBS, but many people can tolerate it if they eat it with other foods.

Meat, poultry, and beans. High-fat meats may aggravate your IBS symptoms. Many people with IBS find that they feel better if they avoid high-fat red meat like prime rib or expensive cuts of steak. Different types of beans such as kidney beans, black beans, and refried beans may cause gas and bloating.

Miscellaneous. Coffee is a problem for many people with IBS. Beer, wine, and hard liquor can also trigger symptoms. Many people can tolerate some types of alcohol, such as wine but not beer, or do better with one type of beer than another (an ale versus a lager). If you drink alcohol, pay attention to your symptoms after consuming different kinds of drinks. You will soon be able to tell which ones you tolerate.

Please do not let this list discourage you. Very few of these will be trigger foods for you. After you identify the foods that aggravate your IBS symptoms, you will discover that there are many other healthy and delicious foods from which you can choose.

How to Use the Trigger Foods List

When you experience IBS symptoms during this week, we want you to use the Trigger Foods list in addition to your Food Journal. Identify any foods that you ate before the symptoms began and make notes about the symptoms that you experienced on this sheet. If you eat the food again and experience no symptoms, that's also important to note.

Grace has had IBS since she was a teenager. She has known for many years that some foods trigger her symptoms. Each week while she was in the study, she made notes on her Trigger Foods list. She was surprised to learn that she was able to tolerate low-fat dairy products. For years she had avoided dairy, thinking that she was lactose intolerant. Now she enjoys 1% milk on her cereal and in her coffee, cottage cheese on her baked potato instead of butter and sour cream, and low-fat yogurt for an afternoon snack. She finds that ice cream and full-fat cheese always cause abdominal pain and diarrhea.

Grace has also avoided most vegetables. By trying small amounts (about ¼ cup for the first try) of a variety of vegetables, she has discovered that she is able to tolerate carrots, green beans, peas, summer and winter squash, tomatoes, cucumbers, asparagus, beets, mushrooms, and potatoes. Grace is able to tolerate broccoli if it is well cooked and she doesn't eat more than ½ cup. Iceberg lettuce and cabbage often cause bloating, gas, and diarrhea.

She tolerates fruits better than she thought as long as she eats them in small amounts. At this point, Grace finds it difficult to get 4 servings of fruit into her diet each day but she is able to tolerate 3 servings. Cantaloupe is the one fruit that always seems to aggravate gas, bloating, and diarrhea.

For several years, Grace has avoided red meat because she finds that it is a trigger for her symptoms. She was pleased and surprised to learn, however, that she is able to tolerate lean pork and on occasion a small amount of lean red meat.

Coffee can aggravate symptoms for Grace if she is under stress or has recently experienced an increase in her symptoms. She has discovered, however, that she is able to tolerate one cup of coffee with her morning snack if she is relaxed and feeling well.

After several weeks of making notes on the Trigger Food list, Grace identified her trigger foods as ice cream, cheese, raw or undercooked broccoli, cabbage, iceberg lettuce, cantaloupe, high-fat red meat, and coffee on some days. After several years of restricting so many foods that she enjoys, Grace feels like she can easily manage her list of trigger foods.

Likewise, we encouraged Krista (page 38) to make changes in her eating patterns. She began eating a small amount of food every 3 to 4 hours. Once she was comfortable with this pattern, she gradually added other foods to her diet. She was surprised that she tolerated small amounts of foods that she previously believed she was unable to eat. Over several weeks, Krista was able to identify a variety of foods in each food group that she enjoyed and tolerated. After tracking her eating patterns and making notes on the Trigger Foods list, Krista was able to see a relationship between her eating patterns, food, and stress. In the end, Krista identified her trigger foods. They include raw cruciferous vegetables, most red meats, full-fat dairy products, spicy Thai food, and black coffee on an empty stomach. These were most notable as trigger foods just before her menstrual period started and during times of stress at work.

Generally, Krista is now free of constipation. On rare occasions, she still experiences severe diarrhea and abdominal pain. Now she is able to identify several contributing factors. She may limit her diet to chicken and rice for a short time but in general Krista eats a healthy, well-balanced diet.

Krista's Trigger Foods List

Food	Notes
Dairy	
Milk	*Nonfat milk in latte—no problems*
Yogurt	*½ cup yogurt—no problems*
Ice cream	*Severe pain after 1 cup ice cream; severe pain after ½ cup ice cream another day*
Cheese	*Small amount feta cheese on salad—okay*
Cottage cheese	
Sour cream	*Low-fat sour cream—no problems*
Vegetables	
Broccoli	*Raw broccoli salad—gas, bloating, and pain (Maybe onion or broccoli?) ½ cup well-cooked broccoli—a little bloating*
Cauliflower	
Cabbage	*Raw cabbage in salad—lots of gas and bloating and pain*
Brussels sprouts	
Onions	*Green onions in salad—okay Cooked onions in casserole—no problems*
Corn	*½ cup—no problems*
Peas	*No problems*
Potatoes	*Small baked potato—no problems*
Fruit	
Apples	*1 small apple—mild bloating Applesauce—no problems*
Pears	*½ cup pear crisp—no problems*
Citrus fruit	*Small orange with lunch—no problem Small orange alone as snack—pain*
Bananas	*No problems*
Berries	*No problems*

(continued)

Krista's Trigger Foods List (*Continued*)

Food	Notes
Meats/Beans/Nuts	
Eggs	*Scrambled eggs—no problems*
Pinto Beans	
Kidney Beans	*¼ cup on salad—very mild bloating*
Lentils	*½ cup lentil soup—no problems*
High-fat Red Meat	*Small steak—severe pain, diarrhea, and bloating*
Nuts	*Almonds ¼ cup—okay* *Peanuts ¼ cup—mild bloating and pain*
Breads/Cereal	
Wheat	*No problems*
Miscellaneous	
Hummus	*2 Tbsp.—no problems*
Garlic	*No problems*
Coffee	*Black coffee on an empty stomach—pain! Black coffee with mid morning snack and after breakfast—usually okay. Coffee can cause pain if work is stressful—even if I have it with food. Latte with low-fat milk seems okay.*
Chocolate	*1 small bag M&M's—pain* *6 M&M's—seems okay*
Beer	*Even small amount causes gas and bloating*
Wine (white or red)	*1 glass either red or white—no problems*
Liquor	
Sorbitol	
Spicy foods	*Thai food moderate spice—pain* *Thai food some mild spice and some no spice—no problems*
High-fat foods	*Small order of fries—pain* *10 fries—pain* *5 fries—no pain!*
Other	

Pay attention to the role of stress in your ability to tolerate food. Many people can tolerate some foods when they are relaxed but the same food can aggravate symptoms when they are stressed.

Keep using the Trigger Foods list for the coming weeks. As you continue, a pattern will emerge and you will be able to identify which foods consistently cause your IBS symptoms. There are extra Trigger Foods forms in the back of the book to use, or you can make copies.

Trigger Foods List

Food	Notes
Dairy	
Milk	
Yogurt	
Ice cream	
Cheese	
Cottage cheese	
Sour cream	
Vegetables	
Broccoli	
Cauliflower	
Cabbage	
Brussels sprouts	
Onions	
Corn	
Peas	
Potatoes	

(continued)

Trigger Foods List (*Continued*)

Food	Notes
Fruit	
Apples	
Pears	
Citrus fruit	
Bananas	
Berries	
Meats/Beans/Nuts	
Eggs	
Pinto beans	
Kidney beans	
Lentils	
High-fat red meat	
Nuts	
Breads/Cereal	
Wheat	
Miscellaneous	
Humus	
Garlic	
Coffee	
Chocolate	
Beer	
Wine (white or red)	
Liquor	
Sorbitol	
Spicy foods	
High-fat foods	
Other	

Your Action Plan

An action plan will help you set and achieve goals. As you think about the goals you want to achieve this week, be specific, make a plan, anticipate obstacles, and decide how you can avoid these pitfalls. Here's what Krista planned to do.

 Krista's Action Plan, Week 1

1. This week I will:

Begin eating small meals every 3 to 4 hours.

When will I do this?

Small breakfast at 8:00 a.m.; midmorning snack at 10:30; ½ of my lunch at 12:30 or 1:00 p.m.; second half of my lunch at 3:30 p.m.; small dinner at 7:00 p.m.; small snack at 9:00 p.m.

What obstacles might keep me from reaching my goal?

Not having time to pack my lunch/snacks before work.
No time for a break in the morning or afternoon.

How can I overcome these obstacles?

I will start packing my lunch the night before work.
I will keep granola bars, low-fat crackers, and almonds in my desk drawer and purse.

Krista's Action Plan, 3 Weeks Later

1.   This week I will:

Add one fruit to my diet each day. If this causes discomfort, I will back off to 1 fruit every other day.

When will I do this?

I will add 1 serving of fruit to my dinner each day or every other day. I will start with a few grapes, then try raspberries, and then try peaches.

What obstacles might keep me from reaching my goals?

My attitude and thought patterns are the biggest obstacle. I am afraid that these foods will aggravate my symptoms.

How can I overcome these obstacles?

I will go very slowly in this process. It will be important to remember that I don't have to eat a large amount of fruit and these are fruits I love. It would be wonderful to add them back into my diet.

My Action Plan

1. This week I will:

When will I do this?

What obstacles might keep me from reaching my goal?

How can I overcome these obstacles?

2. This week I will:

When will I do this?

What obstacles might keep me from reaching my goals?

How can I overcome these obstacles?

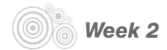 ## *Week 2*

Skills to Build

Food

Begin eating every 3 to 4 hours, starting with breakfast.

Complete your Food Journal each day for 5 to 7 days. Write down all of the foods you eat (including snacks), time that each food was eaten, and amount of food eaten. Describe the stress that you felt and any symptoms you experienced.

Make notes on the Trigger Foods list of any symptoms that you experience after eating any of the listed foods.

Relaxation

Continue abdominal breathing exercise for 2 minutes in the morning and for 2 minutes in the evening.

Continue the quieting response 3 to 4 times a day.

Self-Awareness

Complete the Keeping Track form each day.

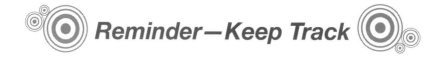

Reminder—Keep Track

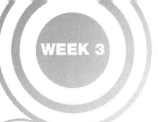

Relaxation Skills

IN THIS CHAPTER

Learn about using active and passive progressive muscle relaxation to decrease your IBS symptoms.

QUICK FACTS

Active progressive muscle relaxation is a form of systematic relaxation. It involves tightening and relaxing different muscle groups in a consistent pattern.

Learning to contract and relax muscles can release unwanted tension and help decrease IBS symptoms.

Both active and passive progressive muscle relaxation teach you to recognize muscle tension and to relax in an effective way.

Active Progressive Muscle Relaxation

An excellent way to develop relaxation skills is to learn how to let go of tension in specific muscle groups. Active progressive muscle relaxation involves identifying and tightening muscle groups, followed by a conscious effort to relax those same muscles. As you tighten and relax each muscle group, you will begin to recognize the difference between tension and relaxation. Once you can tell the difference between tense and relaxed muscles, you can learn to detect and relieve unwanted tension.

This type of relaxation will help you manage stress. Stress activates the nervous system, causing a cascade of changes within your body that often trigger IBS symptoms. Relaxation skills help to bring the nervous system back to a relaxed state. This will positively affect intestinal activity and sensitivity as well as reduce your perception of pain. Many people find that relaxation exercises are effective strategies for reducing abdominal pain and discomfort and for relieving diarrhea.

Perhaps you remember the old song that goes, "The knee bone's connected to the thigh bone . . ." The same concept applies to muscles. When one set of muscles is tense, it affects the others around it. If your neck and shoulders are tense and knotted up, that muscle tension may affect your back and abdominal muscles, which in turn affect your intestinal muscles. When you practice progressive relaxation, you will learn to pay attention to tension in all parts of your body, because it's all connected.

We want you to practice progressive relaxation when you are lying down or sitting in a chair with your head supported. Begin with the muscles in your forehead. Slightly tense the muscles in that area for 5 to 10 seconds while you continue to breathe. Then gradually relax for 20 to 30 seconds. After you have tensed and relaxed a muscle group, you will find that it is more relaxed than when you started.

Andrew, an attorney, has had IBS since college. For the past few months, he has been working to gain a sense of control over his symptoms. He has made several dietary changes and is now working on increasing his ability to relax on a regular basis. At first, he thought he had no time to relax. Eventually he came to realize he might actually *gain* time in his day if he took a little time to practice the abdominal breathing and quieting response that helped decrease his symptoms. Recently, Andrew has also discovered that the progressive muscle relaxation exercise allows him to relax even more deeply.

For several days, Andrew practiced this relaxation exercise at home. Here's how he does it: lying on the floor with a small pillow under his head and another one under his knees, he begins to systematically tighten and relax muscles in his hands, arms, face, trunk, legs, and feet. First, he makes a tight fist with his right hand, focusing on the tension that was created in his hand and forearm. Then he relaxes his hand and focuses on the feeling of relaxed muscles in that area. Next, he gently tightens the muscles in his right hand and forearm, paying attention to the feeling of mild muscle tension. After a few seconds, he relaxes his hand and for several seconds focuses on the feeling of relaxed muscles in his hand and forearm. Then he moves on to the muscles in his upper arm. In a systematic way, he works through his entire body, tensing and relaxing muscles. When he completes the exercise, he tells us he feels relaxed and peaceful.

The exercise helped Andrew become aware of the mild muscle tension in his body. Now, when he becomes aware of mild muscle tension during the day, he uses this awareness as a reminder to increase the frequency of his abdominal breathing and quieting response exercises. The tensing and relaxing of muscles leaves him feeling more relaxed than he remembers feeling in a long time.

Now that Andrew has learned to do the progressive muscle relaxation exercise at home, he is going to find a way to incorporate it into his work day. His plan is to look for an empty conference room with a comfortable chair to sit in so that he can do the relaxation exercise at work. If that doesn't work, he plans to close his office door and turn off his phone during lunch so that he can do the progressive muscle relaxation exercise each day during his work hours.

At the beginning, you may notice that you can't totally relax a particular muscle or muscle group during the relaxation phase. If you notice an area that remains tense, breathe slowly and deeply and tell yourself to "let go of the tension," or "relax."

It takes some time to master active progressive muscle relaxation. Most people can remember the sequence of the exercise after practicing several times. It is important to go slowly at first, until you get the feel of it. The first few times you try the exercise, you may not feel totally relaxed afterward. You will probably notice that you are more relaxed than you were before you started, however. Deep relaxation will come with practice. Once you learn the technique, you can speed up and accomplish deep relaxation in a much shorter period of time.

How to Practice Active Progressive Muscle Relaxation

You can learn to do active progressive muscle relaxation by reviewing the instructions for each muscle group in the chart on page 52 and then practicing the exercise. Read the instruction in the chart several times. When you feel familiar with each position, it's time to practice. When you practice, turn your focus to the feeling of tension created in each muscle group when you tighten the muscles and then focus on the feeling of relaxation created when the tension is missing.

To begin the exercise, sit or lie down in a warm, comfortable place with your arms and head supported. Take a few deep breaths and let your body relax. Close your eyes. Let go of any thoughts from the day and keep your awareness on your breathing. Remember to breathe calmly and regularly throughout

Muscle Group	How to Tense
Hands/Forearms	Make a fist and squeeze
Biceps	Bend elbows, hands up toward shoulder
Forehead	Raise eyebrows
Eyes	Squeeze shut
Jaw*	Clench teeth
Lips	Purse lips like blowing a whistle
Neck*	Push head forward and back
Shoulders	Lift shoulders up to ears
Upper back*	Pull shoulder blades together
Chest	Take a deep breath and hold
Abdomen	Tighten abdominal muscles, pull them in
Lower back	Gently arch back
Buttocks	Tighten buttocks
Thigh	Tighten upper legs
Calves	Point toes up toward head
Feet/toes*	Point toes down and curl toes

*Use caution when tensing the neck, jaw, and back, especially if you have experienced muscle spasms in these muscle groups. Also be cautious when tensing feet or toes, tensing too much may result in muscle cramping. It is important not to tense too hard, but tense just enough to notice an increase.

the exercise, releasing tension each time you exhale.

Begin by tightening your right fist and squeeze hard. Think about the feeling of tension created in your hand and forearm. Hold the tension for 5 to 10 seconds and then slowly relax for 20 to 30 seconds. Focus on the feeling of the relaxed muscle when you release the tension. Can you feel the difference between the tense muscles and the relaxed muscles?

Next, tighten the muscles in your right bicep by bending your elbow and pulling your clenched fist up toward your shoulder. Focus only on the tension in your right bicep. Hold the tension for several seconds and then release your fist and relax your arm. Once again, focus on the feeling of the relaxed muscles in your biceps.

Take a slow, deep, full breath and work systematically through the muscle groups in your body. As you progress through the tension and relaxation process, your body will feel more relaxed. End the exercise by taking a few slow, deep breaths.

Here's a word of caution. Active progressive muscle relaxation can aggravate tension for some people. Those people may find that passive progressive muscle relaxation is more comfortable. Passive progressive muscle relaxation teaches you how to relax your muscles without tension.

Passive Progressive Muscle Relaxation

In the passive form of progressive relaxation, you achieve deep relaxation by focusing your attention on your breathing and systematically relaxing specific muscle groups. As with active progressive muscle relaxation, you follow the sequence of muscle groups outlined above. You do not tense your muscles; instead, you work to relieve any stress already present. As you exhale, let go of any tension in the muscle group on which you are focusing. If there is any remaining tension, release it as you exhale with the next breath. The most important elements of this exercise are:

- progressing slowly from one muscle group to another
- pausing to focus on and relax the muscles passively instead of increasing the tension
- deep breathing to induce relaxation

Everyone seems to have their favorite relaxation exercise. Elizabeth found that she could relax most effectively with a passive progressive muscle relaxation exercise. The active progressive muscle relaxation exercise left her feeling tense and uneasy. People tend to prefer either the active or the passive muscle relaxation exercise. Sometimes, participants found the active exercise helpful in the daytime and used the passive exercise to fall asleep at night. It is not important that you use each exercise in this book. Instead, we want you to practice each one several times so that you can identify which ones work best for you. The goal is for you to have one or two relaxation exercises that you can use to reliably relax quickly and easily.

After several practice runs, Elizabeth discovered that she prefers starting with her head and working down toward her feet. After taking a few slow deep breaths, she turns her focus to the muscles in her forehead. Gently, she lets these muscles relax. For a few seconds, she focuses on the feeling of those relaxed muscles. Next, she lets the muscles of her eyelids and the muscles around her eyes relax. Because Elizabeth carries a lot of muscle tension in these areas, she is off to a good start. It feels wonderful to let go of the tension in her forehead and around her eyes. Next, she lets her jaw drop and releases any additional tension that she was feeling in her jaw and cheeks and in the muscles around her mouth.

When her head and face are feeling relaxed, she moves on to her neck and shoulders, relaxing first the tension that she feels in her neck, the front, back, and sides. Then she lets go of the tension in her shoulders. After taking a few slow deep breaths, Elizabeth moves on to the muscles in her hands, arms, chest, abdomen, back, buttocks, thighs, calves, feet, and toes. When she reaches her toes, Elizabeth feels relaxed and peaceful.

Elizabeth's challenge was fitting this into her schedule. She needed some way to follow through while still being able to carry on with her life. After a bit of practice, she realized that she can use this exercise when she is lying in bed, sitting in her chair at work, or standing in line at the grocery store and even while she is on hold on the telephone. She can lengthen or shorten the exercise to fit the amount of time that she has. Sometimes she just works through the muscles in her head, neck, shoulders, chest, and abdomen. The flexibility of this exercise provides Elizabeth with a skill that she can use throughout the day. Once she was using this exercise on a regular basis, she realized that she was feeling much more relaxed all day long.

Body Scan

You can learn to scan your body to identify where there is tension. To start, get into a comfortable position.

Take a slow deep breath. Your eyes can be open or closed. Focus your attention on physical sensations in your body.

- Is your abdomen soft and relaxed?
- Are you holding your shoulders up by your ears?
- Is your jaw loose, with your upper and lower teeth slightly apart?

Starting at your head, scan your body for any signs of tension. Focus on your body from top to bottom: head, neck, shoulders, arms, hands, chest, abdomen, back, legs, and feet. Notice where you feel or see signs of tension. Repeat the scan, letting go of any tension while imagining each part becoming more and more relaxed.

When the Going Gets Tough

Managing your symptoms of IBS involves making changes in your diet, thoughts, and stress level. Reducing symptoms of IBS may be enough motivation to make a change or give up old habits. However, there are times when making changes can be difficult, challenging, or even overwhelming. You may identify several areas that you would like to work on, but trying to make too many changes at the same time can become unmanageable.

It is important to pace yourself so you don't lose interest or feel burned out and frustrated. If you set your expectations too high, you may feel guilty for not accomplishing what you had hoped and then find yourself coming up with reasons to avoid making changes.

Sarah was determined to learn to manage her IBS symptoms. With great enthusiasm, she began to set goals and make lifestyle changes. At first she experienced a little improvement in her symptoms. Soon, however, she began to feel overwhelmed and had difficulty keeping up with all of the changes she was trying to make. The rapid changes and the discouragement that she experienced contributed to an increase in symptoms instead of helping her to effectively reduce her symptoms.

If you find you haven't yet noticed any progress in managing your symptoms, remember:

- Be patient with yourself
- Be persistent; don't give up
- Don't be hard on yourself or critical
- Problem solve

Instead of giving up, Sarah decided to begin the process again. She decided that she would work on one skill at a time. She began with abdominal breathing. Each day she spent time practicing the breathing. When she was comfortable with the breathing and doing it on a regular basis, she added the quieting response. She practiced this for several days and developed some effective reminders so that she was able to do the quieting response on a regular basis throughout the day. Slowly, she has continued to learn new skills and incorporate them into her life. The pace now was much more relaxed and the outcome positive. This positive response was the feedback that she needed to continue a slow and steady pace to gain a sense of control over her symptoms.

Healthy Thought Patterns

IN THIS CHAPTER

Become aware of your thoughts and learn to change unhealthy thought patterns to healthier ways of thinking.

QUICK FACTS

Your feelings are created by your thoughts, not by the events and circumstances of your day. Sometimes thoughts go through your mind so quickly that you may not even be aware of them.

As you become aware of your thoughts and begin to change unhealthy thought patterns to healthier ways of thinking, you can change the way you feel.

Because your emotional state influences your IBS symptoms, learning to identify and change unhealthy thought patterns can help improve your IBS symptoms.

Cognitive Restructuring

Every day you encounter a variety of situations: irritating (or friendly) people, pleasant surprises, frustrating experiences, tedious tasks. You respond to each situation with your thoughts and feelings, although you may not be aware of this at the time. These thoughts happen quickly and are called *automatic thoughts*. Because they happen so quickly, they often go unnoticed.

Cognitive restructuring means changing your automatic thoughts. This takes a bit of practice but it is well worth the effort. Your thoughts precede your feelings and are actually the cause of your feelings. If you learn to change your thoughts, you can change the way you feel. Feelings such as anger, anxiety, and frustration can aggravate your IBS symptoms. When you learn to identify ways of thinking that are causing you problems and then change the automatic thoughts to healthy thoughts, you can increase your control over your feelings and your symptoms.

People often think that events and experiences are directly responsible for how they feel. For example, if you are late for an important appointment and get stuck in traffic, you may feel frustrated, angry, or anxious. It's easy to believe that your feelings are caused by the traffic. In reality, however, your feelings are a result of the automatic thoughts that are going through your mind.

You might hear yourself saying things to yourself such as

"This stupid traffic."
"I'm going to be late."
"I can't ever get anywhere on time."
"If I miss this appointment, I will probably lose my job."
"By the time I get there, my stomach's going to be a wreck!"

What's wrong with these thoughts? They aren't helpful. You start out criticizing the traffic but end up criticizing yourself and others. They can lead to feelings of frustration, anger, and hopelessness. These feelings have the potential of aggravating your IBS symptoms and making it hard for you to problem-solve and cope with the situation.

With practice, you will learn to recognize problematic thoughts and change them to something more productive. You might replace those thoughts with more constructive thoughts, such as

"The traffic sure is heavy today." (State the facts.)
"I will call and let them know that I'll be late." (Problem-solve.)
"(Deep breath) If I relax, I can handle this situation." (Stay positive.)
"There is nowhere that I can go right now, so I will use the time to do some
    relaxation exercises. That will help control my IBS symptoms." (Relax.)
"Next time, I'll take another route." (Plan.)

These new thoughts lead to different feelings such as competence, acceptance, peacefulness, and a greater sense of control. You have a better chance of avoiding a flare of your symptoms when you take control of your thoughts.

As you learn to change your thinking, you will have more control over your feelings and, consequently, over your IBS symptoms.

Below is a simple diagram that illustrates the relationship between events, thoughts, feelings, and symptoms. An event or situation precedes your automatic thoughts. These thoughts lead to feelings that can bring a change in symptoms or behaviors.

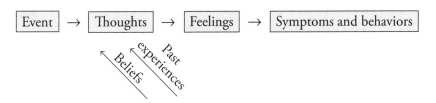

Automatic thoughts go through your mind very quickly. They can be words, short phrases, sentences, or pictures that are influenced by beliefs and past experiences. We will look at the role of beliefs and past experiences in Week 5. This week, you will focus on identifying automatic thoughts. It is not always easy to identify automatic thoughts. Think again about the example of the traffic jam. You may first notice that the traffic is slowing down. Or you may realize you are feeling anxious and your stomach is getting tight and making funny noises.

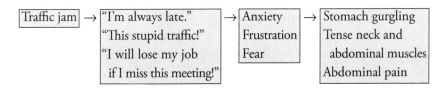

The diagram above illustrates the relationship between the event (traffic jam), the feelings (anxiety), and the symptoms (gurgling stomach). Now ask yourself, "What thoughts are going through my head to make me feel anxious?"

In many cases, you do not have control over the events you encounter. But you do have control over your thoughts. If you begin to quickly identify your thoughts and correct them when needed, you can influence your feelings, behaviors, and symptoms in a positive manner. Your goal is to identify your problematic thoughts as soon as they occur and change them to accurate, helpful thoughts.

In the diagram on page 60, you can see a more helpful response. Changing your thoughts will change your feelings, symptoms, and behavior. With practice you will be able to recognize your thoughts quickly and easily, making changes as needed and gaining control over your feelings and your IBS symptoms.

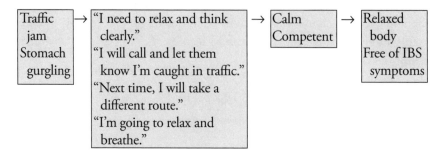

Two Steps in Changing Your Thought Patterns

1. Recognize your automatic thoughts.
2. Change the automatic thought to a healthier, more accurate thought as soon as possible (as in the diagram above).

Everyone has some automatic thoughts that are not rational. These thoughts are based on past experiences and beliefs. In many cases, these thoughts become problems because they influence feelings and symptoms in a negative manner. Many common problematic thoughts have names. Read through the different types of problematic thoughts and try to identify the ways of thinking that are most familiar to you. Identifying and naming your thoughts will help you to see patterns in your thinking. This information will allow you to identify and change your automatic thoughts more easily.

Problematic Ways of Thinking

Do you recognize any of these common problematic ways of thinking?[1]

All-or-nothing thinking. You view things in absolute, black-and-white categories. If your performance falls short of perfect, you see yourself as a total failure.

Overgeneralization of the negative. You view a negative event as a never-ending pattern.

Mental filter. You pick out a single negative detail and dwell on it exclusively, so that your vision of all reality becomes darkened, like the drop of ink that discolors the entire beaker of water.

[1]Cognitive distortions adapted from Burns, David. *Feeling Good: The New Mood Therapy.* New York: William Morrow, 1980.

Discounting the positives. You reject positive experiences by insisting they don't count for some reason or another. You maintain a negative belief that that is contradicted by your everyday experiences.

Jumping to conclusions. You make a negative interpretation even though there are no definite facts that convincingly support your conclusion such as:

- **Mind reading:** You arbitrarily conclude that someone is reacting negatively to you and don't bother to check it out.
- **Fortune telling:** You anticipate that things will turn out badly and feel convinced that your prediction is an already established fact.

Magnification and minimization. You exaggerate the importance of things (such as your goof-up or someone else's achievement) or you inappropriately shrink things until they appear tiny (your own desirable qualities or someone else's imperfections).

Emotional reasoning. You assume that your negative emotions necessarily reflect the way things really are: "I feel it, therefore it must be true."

"Should" thinking. You try to motivate yourself with "shoulds" and "shouldn'ts," as if you had to be whipped and punished before you could be expected to do anything. "Musts" and "oughts" are also offenders. The emotional consequence is guilt. When you direct should statements toward others, you feel anger, frustration, and resentment.

Labeling and mislabeling. This is an extreme form of overgeneralization. Instead of describing your error, you attach a negative label to yourself: "I'm a loser." When someone else's behavior rubs you the wrong way, you attach a negative label to him: "He's an idiot." Mislabeling involves describing an event with language that is highly colored and emotionally loaded.

Personalization. You see yourself as the cause of some negative external event for which, in fact, you were not primarily responsible.

Everyone has some automatic thoughts that are problematic and lead to negative feelings. For people with IBS these thoughts have the potential of increasing symptoms. Which ones do you recognize? Which ones are most common in your thinking?

Cindy felt herself getting more and more anxious as the time for her in-laws to arrive drew closer. "Why did I even think of inviting them to dinner? There is no way that this will go well." (fortune telling) "They are always irritated by the kids, and they never seem to like what I serve for dinner." (all-or-nothing thinking)

Early in the program, many of these incidences slipped by Cindy, making her symptoms worse. But eventually she came to see that there were other ways to look at her situation and faced the challenge of developing new thought patterns. Fortune telling and all-or-nothing thinking were common thought patterns for her, so she was able to identify them quickly and think about accurate ways to change them. "It is true that they didn't seem to enjoy parts of the evening the last time they were here, especially when Jack spilled his milk at dinner and Carrie cried for an hour after dinner. But Jack hasn't spilled his milk for a while, and Carrie doesn't have an ear infection today, so she'll probably be in a good mood. Chances are the kids will do much better tonight."

"Who knows if they will like this chicken recipe? It seems like something adults and children both will enjoy, but I can't know for sure. There is no way that I can tell how the evening will go. In any case, it is an opportunity for everyone to relax and enjoy each other's company. I am going to try to relax and enjoy the evening and deal with whatever the evening holds as it happens."

Changing her thoughts and taking a few slow deep breaths helped Cindy to relax. The feeling of anxiety was replaced with a sense of hopefulness and adventure. Whatever the evening holds, she felt like she could handle it. She noticed that her abdominal muscles were beginning to relax, and the pain was beginning to ease. Maybe this will be an enjoyable evening after all.

You can begin to change your problematic thoughts by identifying and categorizing them. As you see patterns in your thinking, it becomes easier to correct the thoughts. With practice, your new, more supportive responses will become increasingly automatic, which lessens the negative feelings as well as the IBS symptoms.

Using the Automatic Thoughts Form

Take a look at Darren's work on his automatic thoughts. Use the Automatic Thoughts form on the next page to write an example of some problematic thinking that you can recall from the past week. Identify the event, thoughts, feelings, and any behaviors and/or symptoms that you experienced. When you have completed this step, write examples of healthier, more accurate thought patterns that you could substitute and the feelings that might have followed. Table 5 has a list of feelings to help you complete the form.

Darren's Automatic Thoughts

Event →	Thoughts →	Feelings →	Behavior/symptoms
Problematic			
Upcoming dinner and movie with friends	*"I hate eating out. I always get sick."* (*This is all-or-nothing thinking.*)	*Hopelessness* *Frustration* *Anger*	*Considering not going out* *Neck and jaw tension* *Abdomen feels tense, stomach beginning to make funny noises*
A Healthier Response			
Upcoming dinner and movie with friends	*"I am going to relax and enjoy the evening."* *"If I relax, I have more control over my IBS."* *"I will eat a light, low-fat dinner. I will find the restrooms at the theater and sit in an aisle seat in case I need to use the restroom."*	*Sense of control* *Hopefulness* *Calm*	*Go to dinner and movie* *Less muscle tension* *Abdomen more relaxed, discomfort subsiding*

Table 5. List of Feelings

It's common for people to have difficulty identifying and naming feelings that they are experiencing. This list is a helpful reminder of the wide range of feelings we experience. Use this list to identify and name feelings you experience during the week.

Abandoned	Confused	Foolish	Joyous
Adamant	Contented	Fragmented	Jumpy
Adequate	Cruel	Frazzled	Kind
Adored	Crushed	Frightened	Lazy
Affectionate	Deceitful	Frustrated	Left-out
Ambivalent	Defeated	Furious	Listless
Annoyed	Delighted	Glad	Longing
Anxious	Desirous	Good	Love
Apathetic	Despairing	Grateful	Low
Astounded	Destructive	Greedy	Mad
Awed	Determined	Grief	Mean
Awkward	Distracted	Guilty	Melancholy
Bad	Distraught	Gullible	Miserable
Beautiful	Disturbed	Happy	Naughty
Betrayed	Divided	Hassled	Nervous
Bitter	Dominated	Hate	Nice
Blissful	Dubious	Helpful	Panicked
Bold	Eager	Homesick	Parsimonious
Bored	Ecstatic	Honored	Patient
Brave	Empty	Hurt	Peaceful
Burdened	Energetic	Hysterical	Persecuted
Calm	Enthusiastic	Ignored	Petrified
Challenged	Envious	Immortal	Pity
Cheated	Evil	Impressed	Precarious
Cheerful	Exasperated	Infatuated	Pressured
Childish	Excited	Infuriated	Pretty
Clever	Exhausted	Inspired	Prim
Combative	Fascinated	Intimidated	Proud
Competitive	Fearful	Isolated	Quarrelsome
Condemned	Flustered	Jealous	Rage

(continued)

Table 5. List of Feelings (*Continued*)

Refreshed	Scared	Strong	Unimportant
Rejected	Settled	Stupid	Unsettled
Relaxed	Sexy	Sympathetic	Vibrant
Relieved	Shocked	Talkative	Violent
Reluctant	Shy	Tempted	Vivacious
Remorse	Silly	Tenacious	Vulnerable
Respected	Skeptical	Tense	Weepy
Restless	Sneaky	Tenuous	Wonderful
Reverent	Solemn	Terrified	Worried
Rewarded	Sorrowful	Tired	Zany
Righteous	Spiteful	Troubled	
Sad	Startled	Uneasy	
Satisfied	Stingy	Unhappy	

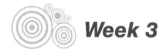 **Week 3**

Skills to Build

Food

Continue to make notes on the Trigger Foods list of any symptoms that you experience after eating any foods.

Relaxation

Continue practicing the quieting response or abdominal breathing 3 to 5 times a day.

Practice active progressive muscle relaxation exercise 1 to 2 times this week.

Thoughts

Write 1 or 2 example(s) of problematic thoughts on the Automatic Thoughts form.

Using the same event, write an example of healthier thinking and the resulting feelings and symptoms.

Self-Awareness

Complete the Keeping Track form each day.

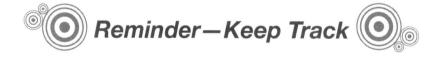 *Reminder—Keep Track*

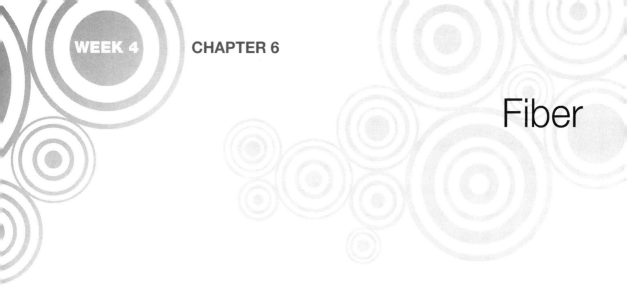

Fiber

IN THIS CHAPTER

Learn about fiber, commonly believed to be a culprit in producing IBS symptoms.

QUICK FACTS

Everyone needs fiber for good health, even people with IBS. Fiber adds bulk to stools. It softens hard stools as well as thickens soft or liquid stools.

Eating a diet that has an adequate amount of fiber will usually significantly decrease IBS symptoms. Most people with IBS need to increase both their fiber and fluid intake. It is important that fiber be increased slowly, with adequate fluid or water, to avoid aggravating your IBS symptoms.

People with diarrhea-prone IBS usually need less fiber than those with constipation-prone IBS.

The Role of Fiber in IBS

Fiber is how we refer to the parts of food that cannot be digested by gastrointestinal enzymes and that, therefore, pass through our digestive track without being absorbed. Fiber is found only in plants; there is fiber in nuts, whole grains, dried beans, fruits, and vegetables. During digestion, plant material is broken down and the nutrients are absorbed. The remainder of the plant material, the fiber, moves along the digestive tract. It adds bulk to stools. Fiber also allows stool to retain water, making it softer and allowing it to pass through the bowel with less pressure on the intestinal walls.

The typical American diet is often very low in fiber: about 12 to 17 grams of fiber a day. You may eat even less fiber than this, thinking that you are preventing IBS symptoms by avoiding fiber. In fact, you might be making them worse.

There are two types of fiber, soluble and insoluble. Most fiber-containing foods have a mixture of soluble and insoluble fiber. Soluble fiber becomes a gel when it comes in contact with water. It makes stomach contents less watery and helps slow the passage of food from the stomach into the small intestine. Insoluble fiber remains intact throughout the intestines, providing bulk to stools. Both types of fiber promote soft, bulky stools for proper elimination.

Some sources of fiber are difficult for people with IBS to tolerate because they tend to cause increased gas or diarrhea. Because of this, you might be tempted to avoid fiber in your diet. However, we want you to choose from the many types of high-fiber foods that do not increase your IBS symptoms. Each of you is different, so you may need to experiment with different types of foods and how you prepare them to see what you can eat most comfortably.

How Much Fiber?

Eating a diet that has an adequate amount of fiber will usually decrease IBS symptoms. The American Dietetic Association recommends a daily intake of 20 to 35 grams of fiber for adults.

The amount of fiber you need depends on the type of IBS symptoms you experience. If you have constipation-prone IBS, you may find that eating 25 grams of fiber or more per day helps you achieve more comfortable, regular bowel movements. If you are prone to diarrhea, you may find that about 20 grams of fiber each day will help add bulk and firm up your stools. If your symptoms alternate between periods of diarrhea and constipation, you'll need to adjust the amount of fiber you eat accordingly.

What Foods Have Fiber?

Fruits, vegetables, dry beans, nuts, and grains contain fiber. There is no fiber in meat, eggs, dairy, or fats.

Generally, whole grains contribute the greatest amount of fiber to the American diet and are easily tolerated by most people with IBS. Because of this, adding a slice of whole wheat bread to a meal each day can be an easy way to begin increasing your fiber intake. It may be surprising to find that whole wheat breads often have more fiber than multigrain products.

We want you to get in the habit of reading food labels so you can calculate your fiber intake. The food label, or Nutrition Facts panel, is very useful. Below is an example food label taken from the FDA's Web article "The Food Label" (www.cfsan.fda.gov/~dms/fdnewlab.html). Note that, in this example, the package contains 4 servings of the food, the serving size is ½ cup, and each serving provides 3 grams of fiber.

When you go to the grocery store this week, read the Nutrition Facts to determine the amount of fiber in each serving. If you are not usually the shopper in your household, take some time this week to go to a grocery store. Look at the Nutrition Facts of the foods you are already eating at home. Then compare the fiber content of those foods to others in the same food group. Be sure to note the size of the serving required to get that amount of fiber. Begin choosing breads, rolls, crackers, pasta, and grains with higher amounts of fiber. Instead of white rice and refined pasta, choose brown rice and whole-wheat pasta occasionally; consider mixing the two types to gradually get used to the new taste. Also, try incorporating in your meals some less common grains, such as whole wheat couscous, bulgur wheat, amaranth, millet, and quinoa.

Look at the food labels on cereal. The amount of fiber found in cereal varies widely. Cereals that contain only wheat bran will be high in fiber but may be difficult to tolerate. Consider adding a small amount of bran flakes (⅛ to ¼ cup) to another cereal that you enjoy. Look for cereals that are low in sugar (less than 10 grams per serving) and contain whole grains.

Fiber is also found in fruits and vegetables. Whole foods usually do not have nutrition fact labels to tell you how much fiber they contain. Use Table 6 to calculate the amount of fiber you are getting from fruits, vegetables, and other

Nutrition Facts

Serving Size 1/2 cup (114g)
Servings Per Container 4

Amount Per Serving

Calories 90   Calories from Fat 30

	% Daily Value*
Total Fat 3g	5%
Saturated Fat 0g	0%
Cholesterol 0mg	0%
Sodium 300mg	13%
Total Carbohydrate 13g	4%
Dietary Fiber 3g	12%
Sugars 3g	
Protein 3g	

Vitamin A 80%	•	Vitamin C 60%
Calcium 4%	•	Iron 10%

*Percent Daily Values are based on a 2,000 calorie diet. Your daily values may be higher or lower depending on your calorie needs.

	Calories:	2,000	2,500
Total Fat	Less than	65g	80g
Sat Fat	Less than	20g	25g
Cholesterol	Less than	300mg	300mg
Sodium	Less than	2,400mg	2,400mg
Total Carbohydrate		300g	375g
Dietary Fiber		25g	30g

Calories per gram:
Fat 9 • Carbohydrate 4 • Protein 4

Table 6. Fiber Content of Common Foods

Bread, Muffins, Tortillas	Amount	Calories	Fiber (grams)
Bagel	1 whole	150	1
Cornbread	1 slice, 2.5 × 2.5 × 1.75 inches	152	1.9
Cracked wheat, 7-grain, mixed grain, oat bran, or whole-grain bread	1 slice	65–70	1.4–1.7
English muffin, white	½ muffin	67	0.8
English muffin, whole wheat	½ muffin	63	1.3
French bread	1 slice, 4 × 2.5 × 1.75 inches	175	1.9
Muffin, blueberry	1 2-oz. muffin	158	1.5
Muffin, bran	1 2-oz. muffin	150	4.0
Raisin bread	1 slice	71	1.1
Rye bread	1 slice	83	1.9
Tortilla, corn	6-inch diameter	58	1.4
Tortilla, flour	6-inch diameter	104	1.1
Wheat berry bread	1 slice	65	1.1
White bread	1 slice	67	0.6
Whole wheat bread	1 slice	69	1.9
Whole wheat pita	6½-inch diameter	170	4.7
Fruit	**Amount**	**Calories**	**Fiber (grams)**
Apple	1 medium	80	4
Apple, dehydrated	¼ cup	52	1.9
Applesauce, unsweetened	½ cup	55	1.5
Apricots, raw	3 medium	50	3
Banana	1 medium, 7–8 inches long	105	2.7
Blueberries, fresh	½ cup	41	3.0
Cherries, fresh	½ cup	42	1.4
Cranberries, fresh	½ cup	41	1.2
Dates	5	117	3
Figs, dried	¼ cup	93	3.8
Grapes, raw	1 cup	60	0.7
Honeydew melon	1/8 of 7-inch diameter melon	56	1.0
Kiwi	1 whole	50	2.5

Table 6. Fiber Content of Common Foods (*Continued*)

Fruit	Amount	Calories	Fiber (grams)
Mango	½ medium	70	1.0
Orange	1 medium	62	3.1
Papaya	½ medium	70	2
Pear, Bartlett	1 medium	98	4.0
Pear halves, canned	½ cup	72	2.0
Peach	1 medium	42	2.0
Pineapple	2 slices	70	1.0
Plums	2 each	73	2.0
Raisins	½ cup	217	2.7
Raspberries, fresh	½ cup	30	4.0
Strawberries, fresh, whole	½ cup	22	1.7
Watermelon, diced	½ cup	23	0.3
Cold Cereals	**Amount**	**Calories**	**Fiber (grams)**
All-Bran	1 cup	160	20
Bran Chex	1 cup	156	8
Cheerios	1 cup	84	2
Corn Bran	1 cup	120	6
Corn Chex	1 cup	110	<1
Corn Flakes	1 cup	100	1
Cracklin' Oat Bran	1 cup	252	8
40% Bran Flakes	1 cup	120–150	7–9
Frosted Mini Wheats	1 cup	170	5
Grape Nuts	1 cup	196	5
Heartland Natural with Raisins	1 cup	468	6
Honey Nut Cheerios	1 cup	126	2
Life	1 cup	167	3
Nature Valley Granola	1 cup	510	7
Product 19	1 cup	110	1
Raisin Bran	1 cup	170–200	8
Rice Krispies	1 cup	110	<1
Shredded Wheat	1 cup	154	4
Total	1 cup	140	4

(continued)

Table 6. Fiber Content of Common Foods (*Continued*)

Hot Cereals	Amount	Calories	Fiber (grams)
Amaranth	1 cup cooked	251	5.2
Corn grits	1 cup	145	<1
Cream of wheat	1 cup	129	1
Oatmeal	1 cup	145	4
Pasta, Rice, and Grains (cooked)	Amount	Calories	Fiber (grams)
Couscous	½ cup	88	1.1
Couscous, whole wheat	½ cup	210	7
Barley, pearl	½ cup	97	3
Bulgur, cracked wheat	½ cup	112	4.5
Macaroni, elbow noodles	½ cup	110	1.3
Macaroni, elbow noodles, whole wheat	½ cup	88	2
Millet	½ cup cooked	103	1.2
Orzo, whole wheat	½ cup	128	6
Quinoa	½ cup cooked	110	2.6
Rice, brown	½ cup cooked	108	2
Rice, white enriched	½ cup cooked	103	0.3
Rice, wild	½ cup	83	1.5
Spaghetti pasta	½ cup cooked	110	1.3
Spaghetti pasta, whole wheat	½ cup cooked	87	3.2
Vegetables	Amount	Calories	Fiber (grams)
Artichoke	1 medium, boiled	64	10
Asparagus	½ cup, cooked	20	1
Avocado	1 whole	322	8
Beans, snap or green	½ cup, raw	22	2
Beets	½ cup, cooked	37	2
Broccoli florets	1 cup raw	63	4
Broccoli spears	½ cup, frozen, cooked	22	2
Brussels sprouts	½ cup, cooked	32	2
Cabbage	½ cup, shredded	8	0.4
Carrots, baby	½ cup	14	1
Cauliflower	½ cup, cooked	14	2
Celery	12-inch stalk	10	1

Table 6. Fiber Content of Common Foods (*Continued*)

Vegetables (con't)	Amount	Calories	Fiber (grams)
Chard, Swiss	½ cup, cooked	18	2
Corn, canned	½ cup	67	2
Corn, frozen	½ cup	53	2
Cucumber	½ cup, raw	8	0.3
Edamame	½ cup	95	4
Green beans	½ cup	22	2
Kale	½ cup	18	1.3
Lettuce	1 leaf	4	0.3
Mushrooms, raw	½ cup	9	0.5
Mushrooms, canned	½ cup	20	2
Onions	⅛ cup	23.5	0.75
Peas, green, frozen	½ cup	63	4
Peas and carrots	½ cup, frozen, cooked	39	3
Pepper, green	1 medium	24	2
Potato, flesh and skin	1 medium, baked	220	5
Potato, mashed, homemade	½ cup	113	2
Potato, French fries	10 strips, fried	101	2
Snow peas	½ cup	35	2
Spinach	½ cup, chopped, frozen, cooked	22	3
Spinach	1 cup, raw	37	1
Squash, summer	½ cup slices, raw	18	1
Squash, winter	½ cup baked	74	5
Sweet potato	Baked in skin, peeled, 5 × 2 inches	117	3.4
Tomato, fresh	1 medium whole	26	1.4
Turnip	½ cup	17	2
Nuts and Beans	**Amount**	**Calories**	**Fiber (grams)**
Almonds	¼ cup, whole, blanched	211	4
Brazil nuts	1 oz. (2 nuts)	184	2
Peanut butter	2 Tbsp.	188	2
Cashews	1 oz. (18 nuts)	165	0.9
Peanuts	¼ cup, dried, salted	214	3

(continued)

Table 6. Fiber Content of Common Foods (*Continued*)

Nuts and Beans (con't)	Amount	Calories	Fiber (grams)
Pistachios	¼ cup, dry roasted, shelled	194	3.5
Pecan halves, dried	¼ cup	185	3
Walnuts	¼ cup, shelled	196	2
Black beans	½ cup, cooked	114	7
Chili with beans	1 cup, canned	324	7
Garbanzo beans	½ cup	110	4
Pork and beans	½ cup	124	6
Peas, black-eyed	½ cup, cooked	100	6
Peas, dried, green, split	½ cup	116	8
Pinto beans	½ cup, cooked	116	7
Snack Foods, Crackers	**Amount**	**Calories**	**Fiber (grams)**
Cheese crackers	10 each	50	<1
Corn chips	1 oz.	140	1
Popcorn, microwave, low fat	1 cup	25	1
Potato chips	1 oz.	155	1.2
Pretzels	1 oz.	110	1
Rye crackers	2 each	73	5
Saltines	5 each	50	<1
Whole wheat crackers	5 each	50	2

foods. These are estimates of the amount of fiber in the foods listed. Some foods with food labels are also on this list. It is always most accurate to read the food label. For example, you may eat a slice of whole wheat bread that contains 3 grams of fiber. This chart lists a slice of whole wheat bread as having 1.9 grams of fiber. That is because the chart takes an average of several popular brands of whole wheat bread. So, use the food label if it is available.

If you are interested in a food that is not in Table 6 and has no label, you can easily look it up on the Internet. For example, if you want to find the amount of fiber in the water chestnuts that you had when you went out for dinner last night, you can search for "water chestnuts nutritional facts," then click on "Nutritional Facts and Analysis" for water chestnuts. You can bring up a nutritional facts label and see that ½ cup of water chestnuts contains 60 calories and 2 grams of fiber.

If you switch to whole wheat (or other whole-grain) products and eat the recommended amount of fruits and vegetables each day, you will probably get sufficient fiber in your diet.

Important Notes

As you increase the amount of fiber in your diet, it is important to increase it gradually. Rapid changes in fiber intake can aggravate your IBS symptoms, increasing pain, gas, or bloating. This does not mean that you cannot eat fiber. But you may be making changes too quickly. If you find that your symptoms begin to increase with additional fiber, decrease your fiber intake to a level that you are able to tolerate and then make any further increases more slowly. The other important action is to increase your water intake, because fiber requires water to do its job.

Fiber mixes with water and other fluids that you drink to form a gel. For fiber to be effective, it is essential that you drink enough water. Set a goal of drinking 6 to 8 cups (48–64 ounces) of water every day. Some people find that they are able to keep track of their water intake by filling a large water bottle and refilling it as needed during the day.

Tracking Your Fiber Intake

Look at the Food Journal that you kept in Week 2 and determine how much fiber you ate each day. The list in Table 6 and Nutrition Facts will help you with this. See Jill's Sample Food Journal for Week 4.

Jill has suffered with constipation and abdominal pain for many years. Initially, she consumed about 12 grams of fiber a day.

In the first several weeks of the study, she tried to make changes in her diet. But this was hard. She was used to preparing certain foods, and she started asking too much of herself too quickly. We recommended that instead she increase her fiber very slowly. Only once did she feel that the increase in fiber caused pain and bloating. With practice, Jill discovered several strategies that helped her keep her fiber intake at an adequate amount without daily calculations. Eating a fiber-rich breakfast was a key factor for Jill. On busy mornings, she had either oatmeal with fruit or a piece of whole wheat toast with peanut butter and sliced banana on top. Each of these contained about a quarter to a third of her fiber for the day.

Jill put fiber-rich snacks in her desk drawer at work, in her purse, and in her glove compartment in the car. She experimented with dry cereals and found two high-fiber, low-fat cereals that she enjoyed and tolerated. Often she would mix a ½ cup of cereal, a few almonds, and some dried cranberries in a zip-lock bag for her snack in the middle of the afternoon.

Salads are one of Jill's favorite meals. She enjoys them for lunch but was surprised to learn that often they contained very little fiber. So she began adding a ¼ cup or a ½ cup of 2 or 3 fruits or vegetables and ¼ cup of garbanzo beans to the greens, along with a few nuts sprinkled over the top. This allowed Jill to continue eating salads for lunch and have a fiber-rich meal at the same time.

Jill also began experimenting with a variety of grains. She found that she didn't like whole wheat pastas but was surprised at how she enjoyed whole wheat couscous. It was tasty and easy to prepare. Adding a little dried fruit and nuts gave it a different twist and even more fiber. Bulgur was another surprise. Jill experimented with different seasonings and chopped vegetables. Adding sage, thyme, chopped onions, red peppers, and broccoli soon became her favorite.

With practice, Jill began to find many quick, easy ways to add fiber to each meal and snack that she ate. These changes made a significant impact on her symptoms, and she was thrilled with the freedom that she felt as her symptoms decreased.

Jill's Food Journal with Fiber Count

Date   *Wednesday, March 2*

Time	Symptoms	Stress level	Food	Fiber
7:00 a.m.		0	1 cup oatmeal	4
			Tea	
10:30		1	1 medium banana	2.7
1:00 p.m.		0	Salad:	
			1 ½ cups spinach leaves	1.5
			1 small carrot, shredded	1.5
			½ cup strawberries	1.7
			⅛ cup almond slices	2
			1 Tbsp. raspberry dressing	
			1 small whole wheat roll with 1 tsp. butter	1.9
4:00		0	2 tbsp. hummus	2
			6 whole wheat crackers	3
6:30		0	½ cup cooked brown rice	2
			Stir fry:	
			¼ cup cooked chicken	
			¼ cup snow peas	1
			½ cup zucchini pieces	1
			¼ cup carrots, chopped	0.5
9:00	B-1	0	Brownie: 1-inch square	
			Total fiber	26.8

Fruit (☑ ☑ ☑ ☐) ☐ ☐ Vegetables (☑ ☑ ☑ ☑ ☑) ☐ ☐ ☐ Grains (☑ ☑ ☑ ☑ ☑) ☐ ☐ ☐ ☐
Dairy (☐ ☐ ☐) ☐ ☐ Meats and Beans ☑ ☑ ☐ ☐ ☐ ☐ 8 oz. of water ☑ ☑ ☑ ☑ ☑ ☐ ☐ ☐
Symptoms: P, abdominal pain or cramping; D, diarrhea; C, constipation; B, bloating.
Rate pain and stress: 1 = mild; 2 = moderate; 3 = severe.

Take a few minutes to determine what you will do this week to begin getting your fiber and water intake to a healthy level. Your plan may look something like this:

- This week, I will go to the grocery store to read labels for fiber content. I will buy some whole wheat bread, some fruit, and some vegetables to have handy at home.
- I will shop on Tuesday after work.
- This week, I will replace the white bread that I eat with whole wheat bread.
- I will do this each day at lunch. I will take a sandwich on whole wheat bread.

Problem Solving

IN THIS CHAPTER

Learn practical ways to solve problems to decrease your stress and IBS symptoms.

QUICK FACTS

Problem solving helps you take control of your circumstances, increase your choices, and decrease your stress.

Because stress may increase IBS symptoms, learning to problem solve can be an effective way of managing your symptoms.

Problem solving involves six steps:

- Define the problem
- Brainstorm the possible solutions
- Evaluate each solution
- Pick the best solution
- Put this solution into action
- Evaluate the results

Principles of Problem Solving

Sharon is a 34-year-old working mother. She is married and has two young daughters who are 2 and 4 years old. Sharon works in the accounting department of a small local business. She has had IBS for the past 10 years and, on a daily basis, experiences abdominal pain and diarrhea. Her accounting job is a busy one but she is able to rush to the bathroom when she needs to. Once Sharon finishes her day at work, she hurries home to fix dinner for her family. After dinner, she works on the laundry, straightens up the house, spends time with her husband and the girls, and gets the girls into bed. Sharon's husband Tim is supportive and helpful. Even with his help, however, Sharon finds that she is exhausted by the end of each day. At this point in her life, Sharon feels as though there is no time for herself. She is surrounded by people all day long. She enjoys her job and loves her family but she longs for some time by herself. To Sharon, this seems like an unsolvable problem that she just has to put up with.

People encounter problems, large and small, every day. Whenever you encounter a problem, there are two ways you can respond: you can problem solve or you can simply react without thinking. A reaction is an impulsive, unplanned behavior that you hope will stop the problem. Sometimes, as when you swat at a mosquito or spit out food that tastes rotten, your instinctive reaction is self-protective and makes sense. Most of the time, reacting to problems instead of problem solving will not improve your situation. It often will make it even worse.

Problem solving involves several steps. First, you define the problem and decide what your alternatives are. Then, you choose the best solution and take action to solve the problem. Finally, you evaluate the solution you chose and make any necessary changes. Problem solving requires that you take time to think. This helps you to respond to problems thoughtfully, in a calm way, instead of impulsively. It is best to step away from difficult situations so you can calm your mind without interruptions. Even when you need to make a quick decision, however, you can use the problem-solving steps. It takes practice and patience to learn to problem solve instead of react, but it is well worth the effort.

There are problems that seem insurmountable such as divorce, major illness, or loss of a job. If you take a big problem and break it down into several smaller pieces, it is easier to find solutions. For example, divorce may result in a move, less income, and changes in child care. By tackling each piece separately, the problem of divorce becomes more manageable, and solutions are easier to find.

Some problems are too big to solve without help. A supportive friend, family member, therapist, clergy, or counselor can help you assess the situation and brainstorm possible solutions. They can support you while you act on your decisions and then help you evaluate your success.

Seeing Problems as Challenges

If you view a problem as a threat, your level of stress increases and you will tend to react with a "fight-or-flight" response. By viewing the problem as a challenge, or a situation that you can manage, you can approach it more calmly and rationally. You'll have a much better chance of solving the problem. Sometimes, all our problem-solving efforts are not enough to totally resolve the situation. Even if solutions cannot be found, problem solving helps you take control of the situation, increase your choices, and decrease stress. It is better to try than to simply give in.

Basics of Problem Solving

Define the problem. Write it down. Be specific. Try breaking the problem into several pieces. Think about your goals. What would you like to see happen?

Brainstorm all possible solutions. Be creative with ideas. Come up with as many options as possible. Ask yourself what others would do. There are no bad ideas. In fact, outrageous options may help you identify possibilities that you were not otherwise able to see. Do not critique the options at this point. The goal is to develop a long list of possibilities.

Evaluate each solution. Now is the time to consider the pros and cons of each possibility on the list. Cross off the solutions that seem unreasonable or out of line with your values. Then list the pros and cons of each. Consider making changes in some options to make them more acceptable.

Pick the best solution. Choose the one solution that you would like to try first. List specific steps you need to take to put the solution into action. Rehearse strategies and behaviors involved in carrying out the solution.

Put the solution into action. You may need to try the solution more than once to know if it is an acceptable approach to the problem.

Evaluate the results. Finally, take time to evaluate the results of the solution. Did you achieve your goal? Are you satisfied with the results? If not, return to the list of options that you created. Choose another option and try again.

Problem-Solving Sample

Here's how Sharon approached her problem of needing time alone.

Define the problem. What is the goal of your problem solving?

I don't have time to myself. There are always people around me. If I am not working, someone always needs something. I would like to have a little time each week by myself.

Brainstorm all possible solutions.

Take 30 minutes for lunch and leave the office. Lock myself in the bedroom for a few minutes after I get home from work. Have someone watch the girls for a little while each week. Go to my mother's house. Take a yoga class.

Evaluate each solution. Consider the pros and cons.

Possible Solutions	Pros	Cons
Leave the office for 30 minutes to eat lunch.	I will feel better if I have time to eat and relax. It would give me a regular time of quiet each day.	It makes it hard on others if I leave the office. They have to pick up my calls. I might be late getting home if I can't get some work done during lunch.
Lock myself in the bedroom for a little while after I get home.	It doesn't cost money. It would be a regular time each day.	The girls don't see me all day. It will be hard on them to know that I am home and won't talk to them. It doesn't really fit my value system. I know that I need time away from the girls, but this would be difficult for them.
Have someone watch the girls for a little while each week.	The girls would be safe. I could really relax.	It doesn't fit our budget. Hiring a babysitter would mean that we couldn't afford to hire a babysitter when Tim and I want to have some time away together.
Go to my mother's house.	I would enjoy seeing my mother.	It takes half an hour to get there. I don't have that much time. I would still need to talk and interact with her.
Take a yoga class.	I would get exercise. I would feel relaxed when I got home. The benefit may be of value for more than just the evening.	It may not fit our budget.

Pick the best solution. List specific steps you need to take to put the solution into action.

I found a class at a nearby recreation center that is reasonably priced. I will ask Tim if he would mind getting the girls to bed on Thursday evenings so that I can take the class. Maybe I could give him some time off on Monday evenings and put the girls to bed by myself.

Put the solution into action.

I began my yoga class 2 weeks ago. (Tim began going out for a run on Monday evenings.)

Evaluate the results. Modify the solution or return to step one and choose another solution if you are not satisfied.

I love my yoga class. I come home feeling relaxed and glad to see my family. Tim also loves having time to run. I don't think that we need to make any more changes now because this is working better than I expected.

Using the Problem-Solving Worksheet

We want you to practice using the Problem-Solving worksheet with a situation that you are currently experiencing. Using the worksheet will help you complete each step. Many people in our study experienced great relief when they were able to recognize that several possible options existed for solving any specific problem. If you have trouble putting your solution into action or find that your solution is not working, remember to go back to your list of options. It's okay to return to step one and redefine the problem, brainstorm some more, and choose a new solution. There are extra blank worksheets in the back of the book.

Problem-Solving Worksheet

1. Define the problem. What is the goal of your problem solving? Be specific.

2. Brainstorm all possible solutions.

3. Evaluate each solution. Consider the pros and cons.

Possible Solutions	Pros	Cons

Problem-Solving Worksheet (*Continued*)

4. Pick the best solution. List specific steps you need to take to put the solution into action.

5. Put the solution into action.

6. Evaluate the results. Modify the solution or return to step one if you are not satisfied.

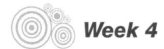 ## Week 4

Skills to Build

Relaxation

Continue the quieting response or abdominal breathing 5 to 7 times a day.

Practice the passive progressive muscle relaxation exercise 1 to 2 times this week (Chapter 4).

Diet

Keep a Food Journal for 5 to 7 days this week. Calculate your fiber and fluid intake each day.

Thoughts

Choose one problem in your life and use the Problem-Solving worksheet to process and resolve the problem.

Self-Awareness

Complete the Keeping Track form each day.

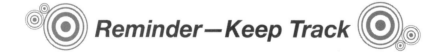 *Reminder—Keep Track*

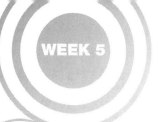

Autogenic Exercises

> ### IN THIS CHAPTER
> Learn another skill to use to decrease your stress and IBS symptoms.
>
> ### QUICK FACTS
> Autogenics is a form of relaxation that works to reverse the stress response and replace it with a relaxed state.
>
> This exercise takes some consistent practice to let your body relax as it becomes warm and heavy.
>
> Many people find that this type of exercise is a very helpful way of managing their IBS symptoms.

Autogenics

Autogenic means "produced by self." Autogenics is a type of self-induced relaxation created by experiencing the sensations of warmth and heaviness. This can be very effective in relieving stress. When you perform autogenic exercises, you can reduce muscle tension and change the blood flow that the stress response induces. This type of exercise generally takes a few weeks of practice, but when you become skilled at it, you will be able to use it in a variety of situations. Many people use an autogenic exercise to successfully fall asleep at night.

Begin by reading through the exercise below several times When you are familiar with the exercise, get in a comfortable position, close your eyes,

Autogenic Relaxation Exercise

Arm and leg heaviness

(Begin with your dominant arm and then focus on the other arm.)

"My right arm is heavy."
"My left arm is heavy."
"Both my arms are heavy."
"My right leg is heavy."
"My left leg is heavy."
"Both my legs are heavy."
"My arms and legs are heavy."
"My whole body is calm and relaxed."

Arm and leg warmth

"My right arm is warm."
"My left arm is warm."
"Both my arms are warm."
"My right leg is warm."
"My left leg is warm."
"Both my legs are warm."
"My arms and legs are warm."
"My whole body is calm and relaxed."

Arm and leg heaviness and warmth

"My right arm is heavy and warm."
"My left arm is heavy and warm."
"Both my arms are heavy and warm."
"My right leg is heavy and warm."
"My left leg is heavy and warm."
"Both my legs are heavy and warm."
"My arms and legs are heavy and warm."
"My whole body is calm and relaxed."

and work slowly though the exercise. Try to visualize the sensation that is being described. For example, repeat to yourself, "My right arm is heavy." Try visualizing your arm as a sandbag that is so heavy you cannot lift it. When you repeat, "My right arm is warm," you might visualize someone pouring warm, soothing oil over your arm or you might imagine the sun gently warming your arm. Repeat each phrase 4 times and then go on to the next one.

As you learn this exercise, begin with the heaviness theme first, then move on to the sensation of warmth. Next, practice combining the two.

Lakeisha, a graduate student with IBS, struggled to learn the autogenic exercise. She had difficulty feeling a sense of either warmth or heaviness. After practicing the exercise a few times, she decided that she would imagine that someone was pouring warm, soothing, tropical-scented oil over her body. When she repeated the statement to herself, "My right arm is warm," she could feel and smell the warm oil running down her arm from her shoulder to her fingertips. It was relaxing and warm! She continued using this picture for the rest of the warmth part of the exercise.

When Lakeisha came to the heaviness part of the exercise, she imagined that her arm was heavy and limp like a bag of sand. Then she could feel the heaviness. It would be hard to move that arm even if she wanted to.

Once she had the ability to feel the warmth and heaviness, Lakeisha found that this exercise was deeply relaxing. It became one of her favorite relaxation exercises. She even tried a shorter version of the exercise. She found that she was able to imagine that someone was pouring that warm oil over her entire body without having to repeat each phrase. She could feel the warm, heavy, and relaxed sensation in a matter of minutes. The exercise was effective when she need a quick way to relax and release tension.

Autogenic Relaxation Exercise (con't)

Breathing

"My right arm is heavy and warm."
"My left arm is heavy and warm."
"Both my arms are heavy and warm."
"My right leg is heavy and warm."
"My left leg is heavy and warm."
"Both my legs are heavy and warm."
"My arms and legs are heavy and warm."
"My breathing is calm and relaxed."
"My whole body is calm and relaxed."

Cool forehead

"My right arm is heavy and warm."
"My left arm is heavy and warm."
"Both my arms are heavy and warm."
"My right leg is heavy and warm."
"My left leg is heavy and warm."
"Both my legs are heavy and warm."
"My arms and legs are heavy and warm."
"My breathing is calm and relaxed."
"My forehead is cool and smooth."
"My whole body is calm and relaxed."

False Beliefs

IN THIS CHAPTER

Learn to identify your false or inaccurate beliefs and correct them. This will change your automatic thoughts and eliminate negative feelings that aggravate your IBS symptoms.

QUICK FACTS

What you believe influences how you think, and how you think influences how you feel.

Everyone holds some false or inaccurate beliefs that lead to problematic thought patterns.

Certain beliefs such as those regarding perfectionism, control, assertiveness, self-esteem, and your IBS can lead to self-defeating thought patterns.

Origins of False Beliefs

In Week 3, you began working to identify ways of thinking that make it hard for you to approach life in an optimistic and productive manner. As you have focused on automatic thoughts as the source of problematic ways of thinking, you may have noticed that they occur more frequently at certain times or in certain situations in your life.

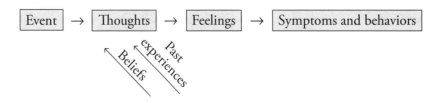

Automatic thoughts are influenced by your beliefs. Each of us has a belief system that influences the way we think and perceive life. Many of these beliefs have their origins in childhood. All young children try to make sense of their world. Children develop beliefs (that may or may not be accurate) and throughout the years collect evidence to support the beliefs that were created in childhood. Over time, these beliefs become deeply integrated into your way of looking at life. Most people don't identify false beliefs until they become a problem.

For example, Laura was a quiet, shy child who grew up in a home where her family moved frequently. Her father was transferred 7 times between kindergarten and her high school graduation. The process of making friends was difficult for Laura, and leaving the few friends she made was very painful. As a young girl, Laura developed the belief that *caring is too great a risk to take.* Each time her family moved, she collected more evidence to support her belief. In high school, Laura began dating Eric and quickly fell in love. After a few months, Eric became interested in someone else and broke off the relationship. She had more evidence to support her new belief that, like caring, *love is too great a risk to take.*

As a young adult with IBS, Laura found that the belief *love is too great a risk to take* influenced her thinking, her feelings, and consequently her IBS symptoms. She enjoyed her job in a research lab, but she had few friends. She often felt lonely and isolated. Her coworkers frequently went out to movies or baseball games together or got together for a barbeque at someone's house after work. They often invited Laura to join them. Remembering the painful process of making, ending, and losing friendships in the past, Laura was hesitant to accept these invitations. She knew that these relationships would not last (fortune telling). She felt anxious and tense each time they invited her to join them. The anxiety aggravated her IBS symptoms; abdominal pain and cramping set in. The fear, anxiety, and pain kept her from joining them, and she was left feeling isolated and alone.

Like Laura, problematic ways of thinking may be holding you back. Becoming aware of false beliefs is an important step in freeing yourself to look at your life and your future more hopefully and positively.

Common Beliefs That Can Lead to Negative Thoughts

Many of the study participants reported having these, or similar, thoughts, often on a daily basis:

- People must think and behave the way that I think they should. I must try and get them to behave the right way.
- Strong people don't ask for help.
- I should not let others know how I feel.
- It is terrible when things are not the way that I want them to be.
- I must be "super competent" in all situations and never make mistakes.
- The unknown and uncertain are always scary and anxiety provoking.

Identifying False Beliefs

Sometimes it is easy to identify false beliefs. For most people, however, it takes some thinking to uncover the beliefs that shape your thinking. You are probably comfortable recognizing feelings and most of your automatic thoughts by now. This skill will help you identify underlying beliefs. If you are able to identify the feeling and the thought behind the feeling, you can continually ask yourself the question, "Why does that bother me?" You can write this in your journal, think it through, or use the Steps to Identifying False Beliefs form found at the end of this chapter (there are additional blank forms in the back of the book). Each answer to the question, "Why does this bother me?" takes you a step closer to identifying your false belief.

Laura, for example, was aware that she felt anxious when her coworkers invited her to social activities outside of work. Her automatic thoughts were, "I will look awkward and won't know what to say." Here's how Laura began to work on identifying her false belief.

Automatic thought:
I will look awkward and won't know what to say.

Why does this bother me?
It bothers me because the process of getting to know people is difficult, and I am seldom able to connect with them.

Why does that bother me?
It bothers me because once I go through the pain and embarrassment of connecting, the relationships never last.

Why does that bother me?
It bothers me because when I go through the pain of getting to know people and care about them, it is even more painful to have the relationship end.

Why does that bother me?
It bothers me because loving people, caring about people, and connecting with people is not worth the pain that it causes.

False belief
Loving or caring about people isn't worth the risk.

Challenging False Beliefs

Once you are able to identify your belief, how do you go about changing or challenging the belief? You can use the rest of the Steps to Identifying False Beliefs form at the end of this chapter for this process also. Ask yourself, "Is this belief true?" and "Does it serve me well?" Sometimes it is easy to see that a belief is not true and doesn't serve you well. Sometimes it is not so clear. A belief might be a little bit true but not serve you well. The belief *love is too great a risk to take* is a little bit true. Love is a risk—that is true. That it's a *risk too great to take* is not usually true. Most often, this belief does not take people to their goals in life. In general, beliefs that are a little true but don't serve you well aren't worth clinging to. However, it is not easy to let go of a belief that you have held for many years and have a great deal of evidence to support. It is important to recognize that you have been selective in collecting evidence to support your false beliefs. There is even more evidence to support beliefs that are true and life-giving.

Laura did not recognize the fact that she believed that *love or caring isn't worth the risk* until the pain, anxiety, fear, loneliness, and isolation seemed almost unbearable. She has held this belief since childhood, always collecting evidence to support it. Now, however, she is able to look at the belief as an adult. She can evaluate the current evidence and look for new evidence that might lead to a more accurate, healthy belief. Her goal is to identify a true belief that will reflect her values, allow her to live with less pain, and reach her goals in a healthy manner. Laura continued to use the chart to challenge her belief.

Is this belief true?
Yes, the belief is sort of true. I have been hurt many times because I have cared about people. There are also a few people in my life that have not left me, and I am glad that they are a part of my life.

Does the belief serve me well at this point in my life?
No, the belief leaves me feeling lonely and isolated. It doesn't help me make friends.

How can I change the belief to make it more accurate and useful?
I can think back on relationships that have not been so painful. I can look for evidence that might indicate that not all relationships end painfully or prematurely.

New accurate belief:
Love is a risk but it adds richness to life.

It was easy for Laura to see that the belief *love is too great a risk to take* was not always true and did not serve her well. To let go of other challenging beliefs, she had to look at the evidence supporting them or actually showing them to be false. She could see that *love is a risk* but maybe the risk of not loving or caring was even greater. As she began to think back over her life, she recalled her parents' strong and healthy marriage. The risk was worth it in their case. She also realized that moving so often had created a bond of closeness and support between her and her brother and sister. Even as adults, they talked often and knew what was going on in each other's lives. Laura had two close friends from college. Neither of them lived nearby but they remained closely connected. After spending some time thinking about this, Laura was able to collect enough evidence to change her belief. *Love is a risk but it adds richness to life.* This change helped her to think differently about her co-workers. Slowly, she began building relationships. It took time but with practice the anxiety decreased and she was able to make friends with some of her coworkers. As the relationships grew stronger, her isolation decreased. Laura was surprised that, without even thinking about it, her IBS her symptoms had decreased.

You may find that problematic thought patterns occur in specific areas of your life. Next, we consider some beliefs commonly expressed by those with IBS. Identify the areas that you struggle with and think about underlying beliefs and experiences that may influence your thought patterns.

Rethinking Your IBS

Conrad, a computer programmer, developed IBS after having giardiasis, a gastrointestinal parasite, following a camping trip in high school. He didn't tell anyone about his symptoms until he was in college and struggling to sit through a 3-hour evening class. It took several weeks before he got up the courage to talk with his doctor. In his family, people didn't talk about "body functions." It was too embarrassing. Conrad held the belief that *body functions are too embarrassing to talk about.* Because no one he knew ever talked about this, he assumed that no one else ever suffered with these symptoms.

After college, Conrad married Jennie. He told her about his IBS once. She didn't ask questions, and he didn't give many details. Over time, Conrad began to feel resentful about Jennie's lack of understanding. "She should know how hard this is. After all, she is my wife" (should thinking). As the tension between them mounted, Conrad's symptoms increased, and he spent more time in the bathroom. Jennie got increasingly upset that Conrad's time in the bathroom prevented them from leaving the house when they planned, often making them late.

You may not talk about your IBS either. This might come from a belief that *strong people don't ask for help* or that *it is terrible when things don't go the way you want them to* or, like Conrad, *body functions are too embarrassing to talk about.* In any case, these beliefs can lead to feelings of isolation and loneliness.

The way you think about your IBS has a great impact on your feelings and consequently on your IBS symptoms. If you assume that you have little control over your IBS and that the symptoms you experience will never get better, you may feel hopeless. It may seem that IBS will ruin your life. When you expect the worst, you'll always be on guard and are likely to feel irritable and uptight. Thoughts about IBS can lead to feelings of frustration and anxiety in addition to aggravating the physical discomfort of the symptoms. It's important to remember, however, that IBS is not a disease process that will get worse. Although the symptoms often fluctuate, you can gain a sense of control and decrease the frequency and intensity of them by using the skills you have learned.

"I am always sick" is an all-or-nothing statement. It represents expecting the worst. A healthier thought would be, "I don't feel well now but I don't always feel bad," or "I have good and bad days, and on the good days, I feel like I have some control over my symptoms."

"I can never live a normal life with IBS!" is an overgeneralization statement. A healthier thought would be, "Even though I feel lousy today, it's not always like this, and there are lots of positive things in my life."

Think about the beliefs that influence your thoughts about IBS. If you aren't sure what beliefs you hold, use the Identifying False Beliefs form to pinpoint and challenge these beliefs.

Becoming "Good Enough"

Tameca grew up in a critical environment, seldom receiving praise or recognition for her accomplishments. As a young girl, she came to believe that her worth was based on her accomplishments. Throughout her high school and college years, she continued to collect data to support this belief. The competitive spirit of her schools only deepened the belief that she must always excel, never making mistakes and never coming in second. Setting goals beyond her reasonable reach led to increased tension in her life. She began to procrastinate, always dreading the process and unsatisfying results of never reaching her goals.

When Tameca began to identify the impact of this belief on her life, she was amazed. She realized that, as a working mom, she was carrying an unmanageable load. Taking on extra projects at work so that she could excel consistently required extra work hours. Volunteering to organize the school carnival, taking treats for soccer each Saturday morning, coordinating the reception that would follow the choir concert, and getting her children to ballet lessons and soccer practice was taking its toll. She was tired, irritable, and often critical of her husband and children. Her IBS symptoms were worse than they had ever been.

With time and practice, Tameca was able to challenge the belief that her worth is based on her accomplishments. She looked for data to support the possibility that her worth is based more on who she is than on what she does. Over time, she began to see that her husband, her children, and her friends enjoyed having her attention, her laughter, her listening ear, and her creative spirit much more than the tasks that used to fill her days. The operative phrase here is *over time*. It's natural to be comfortable with, and even defend, the beliefs that get us into trouble. It is hard work to give them up and takes careful self-examination, and sometimes the help of others, to do this.

So Tameca began to set goals based on the resources she possessed. The time, energy, money, knowledge, and skills she possessed at the time became the factors that influenced her decisions. She no longer set goals that were an attempt to create her worth. Tameca found that a tidy house was more acceptable than a perfect house, an occasional extra project at work was manageable when she didn't have extra projects at home, and that her husband and children preferred her presence much more than her accomplishments.

These insights helped Tameca work to change her belief and thoughts. The tension in her life was significantly decreased, and she found that not only did her IBS symptoms decrease but she also was enjoying life much more.

Many people with IBS have perfectionist tendencies and believe that only perfection is good enough. They set goals so high that they are difficult, if not impossible, to meet. Perfectionists experience little pleasure in working to achieve their goals because they always find something wrong with the result. When things aren't "perfect," they blame and criticize themselves. This leads to a struggle with self-doubt and negative moods. Because they believe that their worth is based on their achievements, failure to meet their own high standards leads to feelings of shame and isolation from others. These beliefs and thoughts generate disquieting feelings that often increase IBS symptoms.

When you believe that you must be and do everything perfectly, you are sure to be disappointed. It is impossible to achieve perfection. Striving for this impossible goal leads to feelings such as frustration, anger, and low self-esteem, as well as chronic procrastination.

To begin to change perfectionist tendencies, it is important to examine underlying beliefs that lead to this quality. Some of these beliefs might be:

- You must be perfect to be loved.
- You must be unfailingly competent and near-perfect in all that you undertake.
- Your self-worth depends on your perfection.
- If you don't go to great lengths to please others, they will abandon or reject you.
- When people disapprove of you, it invariably means you are wrong or bad.
- Your worth as a person depends on how much you achieve and produce.

In addition to challenging and changing the unhealthy beliefs that lead to perfectionism, you will find it helpful to make some other practical changes. Begin to see yourself as a "high achiever" instead of a perfectionist. As a high achiever, you can set your standards high, but within your reach. They should be attainable with the resources that are available to you. Your resources include things such as time, energy, skill, interest, and finances. Instead of being driven by a fear of failure, allow yourself to be challenged by the opportunity to succeed. Getting to this way of thinking will take some time and practice, but it will reward you with less anger and frustration and a greater sense of self-worth.

Suggestions for Moving Away from Perfectionism

Setting realistic goals and expectations is important in managing stress and controlling IBS symptoms.

- Recognize that everyone falls short of his or her goals at times. Begin to change your response to this. Although it is disappointing, it does not need to separate you from others, require you to blame yourself, or make you feel sad about yourself.
- Look for satisfaction in the *process* of achieving a task. For example, it can be fun to learn to paint, create a spreadsheet, or bake a loaf of bread. Try to relax and enjoy the process of learning the skills you need to meet your goal.
- Let go of rigid standards and strive to be more flexible.
- Begin projects early.
- Be accepting of less-than-perfect performance from others as well as yourself.
- Be confident in yourself and your abilities.
- Recognize and accept negative moods in yourself and in others; everyone has a "bad day."
- Evaluate the task or your performance in light of the available time and resources.
- Enjoy compliments and praise; do not dismiss them or use them as a trigger to find fault with yourself.

"I should have been able to finish all the yard work by now," is a should statement. A healthier thought would be, "I did the best that I could with the time, tools, and energy that I had available."

"I never do anything right! Anyone could have done this job, but I messed it up," is an overgeneralization. A more productive thought would be, "This job was hard for me but I learned a lot and could probably do better next time."

Sharing the Control

Curtis, a supervisor at a small computer graphics company, has had IBS for the past 10 years. He suffers with abdominal pain, cramping, and constipation. He is aware that the stress of work aggravates all of his symptoms.

He knows that if he had a stronger, more dependable team at work, it would decrease his stress and his IBS symptoms. He feels that his staff members are lazy and lack initiative, and that no one takes pride in the projects they are working on. He has tried everything he can think of to make them do a better job. He points out their weaknesses at their weekly staff meetings; he tells them about other people in the company that do a better job than any of them. Sometimes he gets so angry that he yells at them when they fall behind on a project, and he demands that they work weekends to get the project completed.

Curtis works hard but unsuccessfully to control his staff. His need, desire, and attempts to control them increase the anger and frustration that he carries everywhere. Although Curtis believes that his staff members are responsible for the anger he feels, his belief that *I must make them do what I want them to do* is actually the root of the problem.

Some people believe that they should be in control of everything and everyone around them. They spend a great deal of time and energy trying to control people and outcomes that are beyond their control. A sense of safety and comfort only seem possible when they believe they have thought of everything and are prepared. Have you felt overwhelmed with feelings of anger or anxiety when things don't appear the way you believe they should be?

It is important to recognize that you only have control over yourself. This means that you do not have control over

- other people, including family members
- the traffic

- the weather
- social events
- world events

You can learn to ask for things and work toward what you want or need. You can plan carefully or even bully people into doing what you want, but in the end, much of life is out of your control. Instead of trying to fight reality, you will do better if you learn to manage your thoughts and your responses to events. Gaining control over your feelings and your responses, which lowers your level of stress and often helps to decrease your IBS symptoms.

Curtis's statement, "They are all lazy and lack initiative" is an example of overgeneralization and labeling. A healthier statement would be, "We are consistently having problems meeting deadlines and coming up with creative ideas. I wonder what's going on?" Realizing that he cannot control his staff may not relieve all of his stress, but it will allow him to see the situation in a new light and problem solve in a more effective way. In the long run, this perspective has a much greater chance of helping to decrease his stress.

Assertiveness: What Does It Look Like?

Trying to control others often requires aggressive or passive-aggressive behavior. Generally this is not a pleasant or satisfying style of relating for anyone. Assertive behavior is an alternative. It is based on the idea that everyone, including you, has a right to his or her own feelings, beliefs, and opinions. This means that each person is the best judge of his or her own thoughts, feelings, and needs and that everyone is created equal and entitled to be treated with respect. The goal is for everyone's needs to be known and met.

When people lack assertiveness, they may believe that they don't deserve to have their needs met or to be treated with respect. The problem is that everyone wants to be treated respectfully, even if they don't believe they deserve it. Eventually, nonassertive people start to feel angry and resentful; this can be a source of increased IBS symptoms.

Assertive behavior does not take advantage of other people. Assertiveness can be:

- Standing up for your rights in such a way that the rights of others are not violated

- Expressing your personal likes and interests spontaneously
- Talking about yourself without being self-conscious
- Knowing your feelings and being comfortable expressing them
- Accepting compliments comfortably
- Disagreeing with someone in a respectful manner
- Asking for clarification
- Saying no
- Being willing to compromise

Henry worked at a large software company and played on their highly competitive baseball team. He awoke one morning with severe abdominal pain and diarrhea. He decided it would look bad if he stayed home, because last night, his had been the last strike of the game. He could still feel the humiliation. "How could I have done that? If it weren't for me, we wouldn't have lost that game. I will never be able to face those guys again. I don't even deserve to be on the team."

Realizing that his thoughts played a major role in the feelings and symptoms he was experiencing, Henry let his body relax and began thinking of a healthier response. "Making the final strike of the game is miserable. But someone ends the game with a final strike every time we play. We are a team, and the results of the game don't rest entirely on me. No one hits every ball. If I relax and let this go, I can probably get my IBS under control. Overall I played well last night. I will focus on that. I will let go of the strike, and face the next game with the confidence I need to continue playing well."

Henry went back to bed for a while to do some deep breathing and a relaxation exercise, and he began feeling better. He took a hot shower, put on some comfortable, loose-fitting clothes, and left for work. Henry was late to work that day, but he went feeling like he could face the day and his team.

Anna left the Monday morning planning meeting at work feeling overwhelmed. She felt her IBS pain and bloating mounting. How did she end up with so many new responsibilities? Anna thought she wouldn't get all of the work done, even if she worked all weekend. Other people hadn't left the meeting with so much extra work. In fact, she couldn't remember anyone else picking up more than a couple of new tasks that need to be completed this week; several people left the meeting with no additional work for the week.

Anna knew that assertiveness had been a struggle for much of her life. She believed that she needed to make everyone happy, often at her own expense. Recently, she had become aware of the relationship between her lack of assertiveness and her IBS symptoms. She was trying to be more assertive, but it was difficult when the whole team was sitting around the table looking at her. She decided that she would go back to her office, review her list of new tasks, and determine what she could reasonably accomplish in the next week. With this information she would go back to her boss and tell her what she would be able to complete this week. Together, they could discuss how to handle the other tasks.

This wasn't an easy plan for Anna to carry out, and she was relieved that her boss was not angry or disappointed with her. They were able to discuss tasks that could be passed on to someone else and identify tasks that could wait another week or two. Anna left that meeting feeling pleased, because she had taken some healthy steps in understanding and developing her assertiveness.

You become assertive by increasing your awareness of your feelings (review the list of feelings in Table 5, page 64) and learning to ask in a respectful way for what you need. If you, like Curtis, are aggressive in your attempts to control, you may need to identify and challenge the beliefs that shape your thoughts and actions.

Curtis believed that, *people must think and act the way I think they should. I must get them to behave the right way.* His tools for making his team behave the way he wanted them to included guilt, humiliation, and manipulation. Not surprisingly, his staff was not motivated in a positive way by these strategies. Instead, they became resentful and bitter and had no desire to work hard for Curtis or the company. This environment did not promote creativity or timely production. The harder Curtis tried to control his team, the more he lost control and the respect of those who worked for him.

As Curtis began to recognize that he was not getting the results that he desired, he became more open to trying a new approach. He challenged his belief that his staff must behave the way he thought they should. Slowly, he let go of the idea that he was the one who must make them behave the right way. He came up with a more accurate belief: *The work must get done, but there are many ways to accomplish this goal.* Gradually, Curtis began treating his staff with more respect. He included them in decisions and gave each of them more freedom. It took time for his staff to trust him, but Curtis was persistent and didn't give up. As the trust and respect increased, Curtis was able to see that he had a responsible, creative team working for him. They may not do things his way, but their way worked well. As Curtis collected evidence to support his new belief, he was able to change his thinking and his feelings. Anger and frustration no longer motivated his words and actions. One day, Curtis noticed that his IBS symptoms had decreased in both intensity and frequency. He was enjoying his job and his staff and feeling better each day.

Table 7 identifies three interpersonal styles: passive, aggressive, and assertive. It provides information to help you tell the difference between these styles.

Table 7. Three Interpersonal Styles

Style	Characteristics	Feels Like to You	Feels Like to Others
Passive	Quiet Little eye contact Not expressing feelings, opinions, or needs and hoping others will guess what they are	Being taken advantage of, a doormat Anger Resentment Helplessness Poor self-image	Push over Frustration—they can't understand what you want
Aggressive	Loud Pushy Accusing Exaggerated show of strength	Superior Controlling others at any cost Anger Guilt	Threatening Accusing Humiliating Hurtful Want to avoid you
Assertive	Good eye contact Firm voice Direct, honest, considerate of others Expresses feelings, opinions, beliefs, and needs when appropriate and with respect	Confident Able to stand up for yourself Valued Effective	Validated Satisfied with relationship

People who are passive rarely experience direct rejection. Aggressive people feel that they have gotten what they want. However, both strategies are escapes or ineffective methods of relating that create more pain and stress than they prevent.

"I" Statements

"I" statements are an easy way of expressing what you feel and asking for what you need. Here is a formula that will help you do this.

When you _____, I feel _____.

Example: When you leave your wet towels on the bathroom floor after your shower, I feel frustrated and angry.

In addition to stating your feelings, you can ask for what you need. You can do this by adding to the above formula.

When you _____, I feel _____. I would prefer _____.

Example: When you leave your wet towels on the bathroom floor after your shower, I feel frustrated and angry. I would prefer that you hang them on the towel rack to dry instead.

If you use this formula to identify troublesome behavior, you are expressing your feelings and needs without blaming the other person. Blaming statements tend to make people defensive and prevent constructive conversation.

Positive Self-Esteem

A healthy self-esteem is based on the belief that you are loveable and capable. Everyone has both strengths and weaknesses. It is important that you recognize this and do not discount your strengths. If you have low self-esteem, you may believe that you are less lovable or competent than others. These feelings often cause people to be nonassertive and critical of themselves.

Emily had just finished a marketing presentation for a new account. Her IBS symptoms had been a problem for several days preceding this. The diarrhea and abdominal pain caused her to run from her computer to the bathroom multiple times each day as she researched and prepared for the presentation. Her belief that *I am not as competent as the others* created thoughts like, "I will make a fool of myself in front of everyone." She experienced feelings of doubt and fear of being "found out." These feelings led to severe abdominal pain and diarrhea.

Right after the presentation, Emily's supervisor complimented her on a job well done. Thinking back over his words later that evening, she thought, "I know he said that I did well on that presentation, but he says that to everyone." This is a discounting the positive statement. A healthier thought would be, "I worked hard on that presentation. I'm glad that he appreciated my work." Emily might have used his compliment as evidence for building a new belief that would be more accurate and helpful in developing a strong, positive self-esteem.

Identifying Your False Beliefs

Can you identify some false beliefs that you hold? Do they influence thoughts about your IBS, perfectionism, control, assertiveness, or self-esteem? Identifying, challenging, and replacing a false belief with a more accurate belief will influence your thoughts, feelings, and symptoms.

You can find a false belief by identifying your negative thoughts and asking yourself this question: "Why does this bother me?" For example, you might find yourself stuck in traffic and late to an important meeting at work. You may be thinking, "I hate being late." Why does being late bother you? "It bothers me because people will think that I am disorganized and incapable." Why does that bother you? "It bothers me because everyone will know that I am not the person that I am trying to portray." Why does that bother you? "That bothers me because I am not perfect and everyone will see." It is false to believe that you can be perfect.

Choose a negative thought and try this questioning process. You may want to use the Automatic Thoughts form to identify the thought and the impact it has on you (see page 62 for a reminder on how to use this form). There are blank forms in the Appendix. When you have identified the thought, ask yourself, "Why does this bother me?" Continue asking the same question until you arrive at the false belief.

Once you identify the belief, think about the impact it has on your thinking and your life. Is the belief true? Does it serve you well? Is it helping you achieve your goals in life? Many of our beliefs come from our childhood. As adults, we are able to see life from a different perspective and develop a more accurate belief system to replace the false one. How would your thoughts, feelings, and symptoms change if your belief system was more accurate?

Steps for Correcting False Beliefs

Automatic thought:

Why does this bother me?

Why does that bother me?

Why does that bother me?

Why does that bother me?

False belief:

Is this belief true?

Does the belief serve me well at this point in my life?

How can I change the belief to make it more accurate and useful?

New accurate belief:

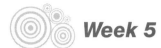 ***Week 5***

Skills to Build

Relaxation

Continue practicing the quieting response or abdominal breathing exercise 6 to 8 times a day.

Practice the autogenic exercise 1 to 2 times this week.

Diet

Continue to gradually increase your fiber and fluid, if needed.

Thoughts

Complete one example of a problematic automatic thought using the Automatic Thoughts form. Go through the steps for identifying false beliefs to reveal the false belief influencing this thought. Think about ways of challenging the false belief and replacing it with a more accurate belief. How would your thoughts, feelings, and symptoms change?

Self-Awareness

Complete the Keeping Track form each day.

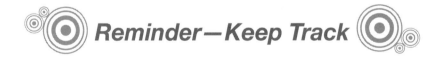
Reminder—Keep Track

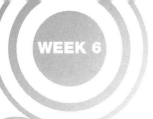

An Effective Approach to Pain Control

IN THIS CHAPTER

Learn about IBS-related pain and your role in controlling it.

QUICK FACTS

Painful IBS symptoms do not indicate that your body is being harmed.

Because IBS typically involves some pain, everything discussed in this book for managing IBS symptoms—your relaxation skills, dietary management, and healthy thought patterns—can work together to prevent and decrease pain.

Visualization is a relaxation skill similar to a self-guided mental vacation that can be effective in changing your focus away from pain.

It is important to use the skills you have learned in this book on a regular basis, or at least at the first signs of discomfort.

Why Is IBS Painful?

Some of the most common and distressing symptoms of IBS are abdominal pain and discomfort. Pain can be caused by altered bowel motility, a heightened awareness and negative perception of bowel stimuli, or an increased sensitivity that may be caused by stress, bowel infections, antibiotics, or small intestinal bacterial overgrowth. We've heard IBS sufferers describe varying patterns and intensity of pain. They may call it aching, cramping, burning, or sharp pain that lasts anywhere from several minutes to several hours. The pain may come and go or remain constant. It may change in type and location over a period of time.

Research indicates that painful IBS symptoms are in part the result of increased sensitivity to pain in the gastrointestinal tract. When there are frequent episodes of constipation, diarrhea, and bloating, the intestinal pain receptors become increasingly sensitive. Over time, this can cause people with IBS to become hypersensitive to normal intestinal pressure variations and experience pain from bowel changes that would not bother people without IBS.

Pain researchers have also suggested many other reasons why people with IBS may be hypersensitive to gut sensations. These reasons can be complex and vary from person to person based on your unique learning history. For example, people who have experienced some form of trauma, such as sexual abuse, may be more "tuned in" to lower body sensations. Or someone who grew up watching a sick relative suffer from pain may have learned to be more cautious about painful conditions.

How you experience pain depends on how you are feeling, emotionally and physically, at the time. Which comes first, emotions or pain? The answer can be either one. If you feel angry, anxious, fatigued, depressed, or bored, it is harder to tolerate physical pain. Sometimes, physical pain comes first, which then leads you to feel frustrated, depressed, and/or anxious. Pain can cause physical changes such as disrupted sleep patterns and increased muscular tension, which themselves increase the level of pain that you feel.

Debra loved her job working in a small, upscale boutique. Recently, she had been taking on more responsibility for ordering, accepting shipments, and setting up window displays. For part of the day, she was the only sales person in the shop. A few weeks ago her IBS symptoms began to get worse. Before this change in her symptoms, she typically experienced pain and diarrhea in the morning and some discomfort during the day. Her symptoms didn't interfere with her work day. Recently, however, she was dealing with increased pain, urgency, and diarrhea during the day also. Once last week she had to excuse herself from a customer and race to the bathroom. Fortunately, Margaret was working at the same time, and she was able to take over the transaction.

Debra felt humiliated to have to leave while she was working with a customer. What if this had happened when she was the only person in the shop? She couldn't leave in the middle of a transaction. What would she do? She wouldn't be able to handle the situation. Debra found herself worrying more and more about this possibility. She was becoming increasingly anxious at work. Whenever she experienced abdominal discomfort, she felt herself panic, tightening her abdominal muscles and bracing against the pain. Her symptoms continued to increase in intensity, and by the end of the week, she resigned from her job.

Our study participants were so conscious of their uncomfortable and inconvenient symptoms that they tended to pay closer attention to bowel sensations than people without IBS. This focus actually made their symptoms worse. They worried about when they would experience gas pain or diarrhea. If they became uncomfortable, they wondered, "Will it get worse? Will it ruin my whole evening?" The more they focused on their abdominal symptoms, the more it upset them and the more intense the level of pain and distress became.

It is important to pay enough attention to your body to know when to intervene, without getting so focused that you become anxious and bring on more symptoms. If you understand what is happening when you experience pain, it will help you feel more in control. It is also important to remember that even though IBS pain can be uncomfortable or distressing, it is not causing harm to your body

Managing the Pain

You have learned the strategies you need to manage your pain. The key to pain management is using those strategies that you have found effective *on a regular basis* to decrease your overall symptoms. Be aware of your earliest pain cues: these may be tight shoulder or abdominal muscles, gurgling stomach sounds, or a slight increase in abdominal pain. When you notice these early symptoms, take action immediately! Use the strategies that will minimize or relieve the symptoms. It may be helpful to leave a tense environment. Evaluate your thoughts. Are they thoughts that lead to feelings of anger, anxiety, frustration, or other feelings that trigger symptoms for you? Many people find that they are able to avoid most moderate-to-severe bouts of abdominal pain by using relaxation exercises. When they notice the first cues that the pain is increasing, they find a quiet spot to sit or recline and spend several minutes doing abdominal breathing or other relaxation exercises that they find effective. Then they move into some of the strategies discussed later in this chapter.

Debra found that she missed her job a great deal. She longed to

Keys to Pain Management

- Identify when you generally experience pain.
- Recognize early pain cues.
- Take action before the pain becomes severe! Use the target strategies you have identified.

be back at work but instead felt trapped at home. For a long time, she felt trapped in this situation. After considerable thought, she decided that she would work on developing strategies and come up with a plan that would help her manage her pain and return to work.

Debra started by doing abdominal breathing every hour or two during her day. She dusted off a relaxation CD she had purchased but never opened and began spending 10 minutes each day listening to one of the exercises on the CD. In the past, she thought that she was too busy for relaxation but now she had more time.

Eating every 3 to 4 hours was an important part of Debra's plan. How could she do this on a regular basis? A roadblock! This left her feeling stuck for a while until she noticed a friend who carried snacks in her purse and car. It was difficult to decide how to avoid the high-fat fast foods—they were everywhere, even as free samples in the supermarket. For Debra, nothing was instant or easy. But she stuck it out and, feeling determined, was able to cut way back on the junk food. With continued effort, she made progress toward her goals.

Reassessing her thoughts was an important part of Debra's plan. She began journaling again. This gave her an opportunity to think about the problematic thoughts that caused her to feel anxious and afraid. She began talking to herself differently.

> "I will keep working on this plan until it is effective and fits the life that I want to have."
> "When I stay relaxed, I can really reduce the pain and the diarrhea."
> "There is no reason to feel humiliated because I have IBS. Many people suffer with this."
> "I am glad that this can be managed with lifestyle changes."
> "I can make these changes and keep them up. One result is that I already feel better."

Debra began getting out more and incorporating these strategies into her life. She started going for short walks. With practice, she learned to keep her mind on something other than the fact that she couldn't get to a bathroom quickly if she needed one. She kept her body relaxed and her mind on the scenery. Gradually, she increased the length of her walks. She began getting together with friends. Locating the restroom, sitting in a spot where she could get out easily if she needed to, being careful with her thoughts, and keeping her body relaxed allowed her to enjoy the time with friends.

About 6 weeks later, she noticed that the usual pain and diarrhea that she had experienced nearly every morning for the past 10 years was almost gone. Debra was able to recognize the tightening of her abdominal muscles and the mild abdominal discomfort that precedes the moderate pain she occasionally experienced. When she becomes aware of these cues, she finds a quiet spot to relax, do some abdominal breathing, and do a passive muscle relaxation exercise. When the pain begins to subside, she calls a friend, reads a good book, or takes a warm bath. The quiet distraction helps to keep the pain from returning. Very rarely does she experience severe abdominal pain, and when she does it is short lived. In fact, Debra realizes that many days she doesn't even think about her IBS. Her strategies have become habits. They no longer require monitoring charts and special attention to her thoughts. She has kept up the habit of journaling because she enjoys it and finds it a useful way to process her feelings and relieve stress.

Three months later, Debra felt confident enough that she wanted to return to work. She began working half days and found that she had no problems with her IBS. Her dietary, relaxation, and thought strategies are still a part of her life. Slowly, she increased her work hours. The strategies that Debra felt she didn't have time for in the past have enabled her to build a life that she enjoys.

So far, we have provided some very effective ways to manage pain: changing your thought patterns, distracting your focus, and using relaxation techniques to calm your mind and body. You can also manage pain by controlling your diet and avoiding trigger foods, especially when you are having a flare of symptoms. We suspect that, like Debra and many other study participants, the pain that you experience with IBS has been decreasing as you have learned new ways of managing your symptoms. However, you may continue to have some bouts of pain.

Reacting to Pain

It is important to stay as relaxed as you can when dealing with pain. If your response involves tensing muscles, bracing against pain, rapid shallow breathing, or even telling yourself that "this will be terrible," a cascade of changes will occur in your body. Your blood pressure and heart rate increase, your muscles become more tense, and the level of pain increases. Instead, we want you to use the pain as a cue to start doing what you need to do to manage the pain. Rather than reacting with anxiety, fear, hopelessness, or any other response that takes away your ability to be in charge, take a slow, deep breath, let your muscles relax, and change your thoughts to something more accurate and helpful.

Begin by taking note of how you respond to pain. What happens to your muscles and to your breathing? What goes through your mind at the first sign of discomfort? The way you think about these first signs of discomfort can lead to a chain of self-defeating thoughts and feelings. For example, perhaps your first thought is, "Oh, no! The pain is back." As quickly as this thought goes through your head, you may tighten your jaw, neck, and abdominal muscles. Your next thoughts might be, "It always gets worse." "Nothing helps." Finally, you think, "I am not going to be able to handle this. I need to go home—NOW." The anxiety builds and causes a cycle of stress and pain. As the pain becomes more intense, you may start feeling angry, depressed, or hopeless, which in turn increases your stress and intensifies the pain you feel.

You have another way of responding to those first signs of pain. Changing your thinking and your physical response is a healthy step toward a sense of being capable of handling your symptoms. When you experience those first mild cues, you might think, "Oh, it is time for me to relax. I know how to handle this. If I catch it early, this discomfort won't get worse." These thoughts lead to feelings of calmness, hope, and competence—feelings that don't have the risk of increasing your symptoms. You can break the cycle of pain by changing your thoughts, slowing your breathing, and relaxing your muscles, using the strategies that you have found to be effective in managing your symptoms.

Changing Your Focus

Another way to get your thoughts in a better place to manage your symptoms is by distracting yourself from the pain and focusing on something else. Remember that the more you focus on pain, the more intensely you will experience it. Ways of changing your focus include activities that take your mind off the pain. Listening to music, doing housework, taking a walk, watching sports, reading, gardening, working on a hobby, or any other activity that keeps your mind occupied can be good distractions from pain. Some people find that walking or other exercise helps relieve gas pain or constipation discomfort. Other people lie with their knees to their chests or take a warm bath to relax. Gentle massage of the painful area can sometimes help you relax and ease the pain.

Avoid isolating yourself. When alone, you are more likely to focus on the pain or feel frustrated or depressed. Talking with someone or joining others in an activity can be an effective distraction.

Try to think differently about your pain. Imagine the pain as simply something going on in your body—just normal bowel contractions, for example. Some people have found that using a more playful image helps. For example, one woman imagined a group of little workers in her bowel, running around pushing full wheelbarrows.

Slowly counting backward prevents you from focusing on the pain and promotes relaxation. Start by closing your eyes and count backward by ones from 100 to 1 (100, 99, 98, and so on . . .). If this is too easy, trying counting backward by 2, 3, or 7.

Listening to music changes your focus and is also a wonderful way to relax. For the purpose of relaxation, it important to select music that is peaceful, soothing, and enjoyable. For distraction, you could choose music that makes you sing along, think, or laugh.

Some people find it helpful to listen to a relaxation CD. When you are in pain, you may find that it is difficult to concentrate. The voice of someone talking you through a relaxation exercise may help you focus and relax more easily.

Relaxation

Calming your mind and body using relaxation techniques is another way of managing pain. When you relax, you break the cycle of stress and pain. Abdominal breathing, the quieting response, active progressive relaxation, and visualization are all effective, not only for decreasing pain but also for preventing pain from occurring in the first place.

If you take time to relax during the day, even if it is just for a few minutes each hour, muscle tension and abdominal pain and discomfort decrease. As a result, pain is less frequent and less intense. As your relaxation skills increase, you will become aware of early signs of stress and pain such as increased muscular tension, shallow or rapid breathing, or cold extremities. These early signs become cues, telling you to relax, using any of the above techniques. This increased awareness of your body allows you to take an active role in managing your stress and therefore your pain. No longer does the pain control you; you control how you respond to pain.

When you are first learning relaxation skills, it is important to practice them when you are calm and not in pain. If you are in pain, it may be hard to change your focus or to stop thinking about the pain. You may try too hard and become frustrated. This makes the learning process ineffective, unrewarding, and discouraging.

Robert was trying to manage his IBS symptoms with relaxation. Every time the pain was severe, he would try to lessen the pain by doing the passive progressive muscle relaxation exercise. It wasn't working. Unfortunately, he had skipped two important steps: practicing when he was relaxed and beginning the relaxation before the pain became severe. We discussed with Robert that his chances of relieving severe pain were minimal but his chances of relieving mild discomfort were excellent. However, he needed to practice his relaxation exercises on a regular basis, before the pain started. Once Robert realized these mistakes, he had renewed energy for practicing. Each morning he spent a few minutes doing a passive progressive muscle relaxation exercise. It surprised him to discover that his consistent practice helped to decrease both the intensity and frequency of his pain. Robert tells us that he hasn't had severe abdominal pain for several weeks and that when he experiences the mild symptoms, he is able to get them under control using relaxation skills.

Some people have a tendency to brace themselves when walking or sitting to avoid pain. When you hold yourself stiffly to protect the part of you that hurts, you overuse other sets of muscles. Bracing not only increases muscle tension, it also takes a lot of energy. As a result, you feel more fatigued and your pain is more intense. When you relax, muscle tension is reduced, the pain is less, and walking or sitting is more natural and comfortable.

An Individual Pain Management Plan

Effective pain management plans will vary. Careful monitoring and practice will help you develop a plan that works for you. Think about when your symptoms generally occur, identify the early cues, and list the strategies you find effective for reducing or relieving the pain.

Debra, the woman who quit her job at the boutique because of her symptoms, developed a very effective plan (page 117).

Melissa's plan (page 118) is quite different from Debra's. Melissa is the mother of two teenage children and has had IBS for the past 10 years. Recently, she has been monitoring her symptoms and working on a plan to get her IBS symptoms under control. The lifestyle changes she has made have significantly reduced her symptoms. However, she continues to experience bouts of moderate-to-severe abdominal pain and constipation for 3 to 4 days before her menstrual cycle begins.

Using her plan, Melissa was able to decrease her IBS symptoms prior to her menses. For the past 2 months, she has had mild abdominal pain and

Debra's Pain Management Plan

My IBS symptoms generally occur:
My worst symptoms happen at work. I also experience them when I am anxious about not being able to find a bathroom.
The early cues for these symptom are:
<u>Thoughts</u>: *"It is humiliating to have to leave a customer or for people to know that I have IBS. I can't handle this."*
<u>Feelings</u>: *Anxiety and fear*
<u>Physical sensations</u>: *Tight abdominal muscles, heart pounding, increasing low abdominal pain*
Actions to reduce or relieve these symptoms:
<u>Diet</u>: *Eat small frequent meals. Healthy snacks at work.*
<u>Thoughts</u>: *As soon as I experience those early cues, remind myself that:*
"I have a plan." *"I can handle this."* *"The plan has worked in the past, and it will work today."* *"When I stay relaxed, I can really reduce the pain and the diarrhea."* *"There is no reason to feel humiliated because I have IBS. Many people suffer with this."* *"I am glad that this can be managed with lifestyle changes."* *"I can make these changes and keep them up."*
<u>Relaxation</u>: *Begin doing some slow abdominal breathing. Let my abdominal muscles relax. Find a quiet place to sit or lay down and do a passive progressive muscle relaxation exercise.*
When the pain lessens or subsides, get my mind on something else. Go back to work, call a friend, or read a book.

constipation prior to her menses but no moderate or severe symptoms. Each month she puts a reminder in her calendar so that she knows when to start her plan.

Debra and Melissa both have pain management plans that work for them. They were able to identify when they were most vulnerable to the pain, what their early cues were, and which strategies would be most effective.

Use the Pain Management Plan forms in the back of the book to write a plan that will work for you.

How Others Can Help—or Hurt

The support you get from those around you can play a role in your pain management. This support can be very positive and helpful. For example, if your discomfort is related in part to your putting unrealistic expectations on

Melissa's Pain Management Plan

My IBS symptoms generally occur: *I have bouts of severe abdominal pain and constipation 3 to 4 days before my period begins.*
The early cues for these symptom are: <u>Thoughts</u>: *"I don't have time for this."* *"It makes me so angry that this happens every month."* <u>Feelings</u>: *Irritation, dread, anger* <u>Physical sensations</u>: *Vague abdominal discomfort, increasing to moderate-to-severe abdominal pain. Constipation.*
Actions to reduce or relieve these symptoms: <u>Diet</u>: *Increase my fiber intake to about 28 grams/day for the 7 days before my period. Drink 64 oz. of fluid during those 7 days.* <u>Thoughts</u>: *Remind myself that:* *"I need to relax."* *"If I take care of myself, I increase my chances of avoiding the pain and constipation."* *"It is easier to take care of myself than it is to suffer with the IBS symptoms."* <u>Relaxation</u>: *Do the quieting response 6 to 8 times each day for the 7 days before my period begins. Do a short autogenics exercise each day for these 7 days.* *Take a walk each evening. Try a warm bath for distraction and to relax.*

yourself, and your spouse or others lighten your load, your anxiety-producing thoughts, tension, and pain may decrease.

However, support can have another, less positive side. It may also *increase* your experience of pain or other symptoms. Here's how that happens. Tim's wife is aware of his IBS. When Tim mentions that he may be feeling symptoms coming on, Lisa, who is a caring and sensitive woman, starts focusing on Tim's symptoms. Throughout the day, she almost constantly checks in with Tim about how he is feeling. This does the opposite of what we want you to try doing: distracting yourself. Lisa's behavior actually makes Tim *more* anxious! He certainly wants to feel well and please her. Like Tim, maybe your spouse even encourages you to not go to work, to rest in bed, or to let him or her do everything for you when you are in pain. We all like this kind of pampering occasionally. However, if this attention encourages illness rather than wellness, research has shown it can lead to a "sick role" pattern that could be hard for you to break. How can you avoid, or end, this pattern?

- Show those around you who want to support you how they can help by asking for what you need such as time alone.
- Ask them to encourage wellness rather than encouraging you to be sicker than you are.
- Teach them skills such as relaxation and distraction, so they can work with, not against, you as you try to apply these skills.

Visualization

Visualization, also known as guided imagery, is similar to daydreaming. It is a relaxation technique where you consciously create a mental picture with a goal of changing how you feel. When you create a mental picture, your body can respond to the visualization as if it were a real experience. This technique is used for relaxation, healing, and managing pain in addition to other relaxation exercises.

Visualization can be done sitting, lying down, or even standing once you have mastered the skill. Read the visualization exercise instructions until you become familiar with the technique.

Most people find this exercise enjoyable and very relaxing. With practice, you can create this mental vacation whenever you need to relax. Create your own special place by using your imagination. The place can be anywhere: a meadow, a hilltop, a tropical island, a forest, or a special room of your own design. Whatever the setting, it should be a

Visualization Exercise

Gently close your eyes. Take a deep, slow breath. Hold your breath for a moment and then exhale fully and completely. Continue to breathe slowly and naturally. Imagine that with each breath you can blow away muscle tension and allow yourself to become more and more relaxed.

Let your mind take you on a mental vacation. For example, imagine yourself lying on a beautiful beach on a calm, warm day. You can see the sandy beach and the clear blue water. In the distance you see a bright sail on a boat as it peacefully skims across the water. Feel the warm sunlight on your face, your arms and hands, your legs and feet, and your abdomen. Feel the soft, gentle breeze. Listen to the rustle of the trees, the waves splashing on the shore, and the seabirds calling. Taste the salt in the air. Sink deeper into the warm, soft sand, becoming totally relaxed and at peace.

Take a few minutes to enjoy this mental vacation. Remind yourself that you can come back and relax here whenever you want. You can stay for any length of time.

Now slowly open your eyes. Take a full, deep breath and stretch. Enjoy the feeling of calmness and relaxation as you gradually return to alertness.

place that feels welcoming, calm, and safe. When imagining your special place, be specific when picturing the surroundings. Be sure to include details involving all your senses: sight, hearing, smell, taste, and feel.

> - What do you see? Look around you and absorb all the sights, the colors, and shadows.
> - What do you hear? Birds calling? Leaves rustling? Wind in the trees? Waves?
> - What do you smell? Flowers? Cut grass? Pine? Freshly baked cookies?
> - What do you feel? Warmth from the sun? Grains of sand? Cool breezes?
> - What do you taste? Salty air? Homemade ice cream?

By using all your senses you become involved in the scene that you create. The image becomes more relaxing and more useful as a distraction.

Ingrid is the mother of three young children, a son who is 3 and twin girls who are almost 2 years old. She has had IBS for about 10 years, and over the past several months her abdominal pain and cramping have increased. The pain begins almost every evening while she is fixing dinner. The children are hungry and often tired. They all seem to need her attention at the same time, while she is trying to focus on getting dinner ready. At some point, all three toddlers end up in tears, and Ingrid realizes that she has abdominal cramping and pain.

Ingrid decided to work on a plan to manage her symptoms more effectively during these chaotic times. Relaxation has been a useful tool for her in the past. She decided that she is going to begin doing some abdominal breathing every hour or two during the day. Each afternoon while the children are napping, she takes a few minutes to do a visualization exercise.

Lying down on her bed, she begins her relaxation exercise with some deep breathing. Then she visualizes herself walking into the woods in a park near her childhood home. She walks along a path that is soft, flat, and well marked. The sun is hidden by the canopy of trees above her head. The muted greens and browns of the evergreen trees are peaceful and relaxing. She reaches out to touch the new growth on the branches of a fir tree; the soft, tender needles are a vibrant lime green. She looks at the lacy boughs and stringy bark of the cedar trees. A huckleberry bush grows out of a dead tree stump, tiny green leaves with red berries. She picks a berry and puts it in her mouth, enjoying its tart flavor. Walking a little deeper into the forest, she is aware of the heady scent of the fir trees and the earthy smell of the soft dirt path beneath her feet. The deeper that she goes into the woods, the quieter it becomes. She hears the gentle thud of her footsteps on the path and the occasional call of a bird announcing her presence in their world. The silence is peaceful. The cool, moist shade is a relief from the summer heat. Ingrid continues to walk, peacefully aware of all that is around her. . . . After a while, she notices an increase in light, a warmth in the air, and the sound of a gentle breeze and becomes aware that she is on a circular path, returning her to her world. She takes a few deep breaths and opens her eyes, feeling refreshed, relaxed, and ready to reenter her world.

The first afternoon that she tried this, dinner time was much the same as others. The children were crabby, they all needed her at once, and dinner was on the stove. But Ingrid was different. She felt relaxed in her chaotic kitchen. She took a deep breath, let her shoulders relax, and reminded herself that this is a phase, the children will grow up, and she can handle this chaos. Later that night, she realized that she was free of abdominal pain and cramping all afternoon.

But the next day, a child woke up from a nap screaming in the middle of her visualization exercise in the forest. Ingrid felt discouraged, as if her goal were impossible. She quit her "walks" for a while. Then she tried a "plan B" and created a plan to have shorter walks for days when long ones were not possible. There are always challenges and setbacks. We want you to expect them and use your problem-solving skills to create a plan B. This will keep you from becoming discouraged. We like to say that changing old patterns is a marathon, not a sprint.

Finding ways to manage your pain effectively may take a little time and some techniques may work better for you than others. It helps to keep a log of your pain on the Keeping Track form, noting the time, frequency, type, location, and intensity of pain. When you monitor your symptoms of pain, you will become increasingly aware of the early signs of discomfort. It is at that point that managing pain is the most effective.

If you encou nter obstacles, you are not alone. Study participants told us they had to overcome many kinds:

- They forgot what to do.
- Those around them were not supportive in either giving the help they needed or in encouraging wellness.

- They received little reward at first for following the suggestions for pain: "I am doing what I am supposed to do. Why do I still have pain?" "Mom, why won't you do everything for me that you used to?"
- They could not figure out how to have the time to do these things.
- They had a plan, but when the time came, they weren't exactly sure what to do: "I said I would take the time to relax regularly, but what does regularly mean?"

You can overcome these obstacles. The solutions for doing that will be unique to you, but others did the following:

- Set up a reminder system.
- Problem solving: Plan ahead. Identify challenges that you might encounter and think of strategies to use when they occur.
- Be very specific with plans and be clear about what you need to do and when; for example, "relax for 2 minutes every hour when at work," rather than "relax regularly."

As you begin to experiment with different ways of managing the pain, use the Keeping Track form to record the results.

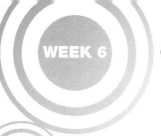

A Healthy Approach to Sleep

IN THIS CHAPTER

Learn about sleep and how relaxation skills and healthy thought patterns can be combined with good sleep habits to help you sleep well on a regular basis.

QUICK FACTS

Sleep affects your mental, emotional, and physical health. Most people need 7 to 9 hours of sleep each night.

Even a brief episode of insomnia can increase your IBS symptoms and lead to a chronic sleep problem.

Your Need for Sleep

Dan struggles to manage his diarrhea and abdominal cramping on a daily basis even when he is rested. When he does not get enough sleep, he has noticed that his IBS symptoms become much worse. Working and going to school has not left enough time for sleep over the past few weeks. When he does finally get to bed, he hasn't been able to fall asleep. His mind goes back over the day, thinking and rethinking about how he might have handled different situations or reviewing ideas for upcoming papers and projects. The longer he lays in bed awake, the more he worries about how little sleep he is going to get and how bad he will feel tomorrow.

Recently, Dan decided to start exercising. When he gets home from school or the library each evening, he lifts weights and then runs on the treadmill until he is so tired he can't do anything but fall into bed and sleep. At first this plan seemed to work well. He fell into bed and right to sleep just as he planned. On a regular basis, however, he began to awaken in the early morning and would lie in bed awake for hours. His tension increased as he worried about the time and how little sleep he would get that night.

Most people need 7 to 9 hours of sleep a night. This may sound like a lot of time sleeping, and indeed it is. It is about one third of your life or, for the average person, 24 years in bed! Do you consider this wasted time or time well spent? If you get much less than 8 hours of sleep per night, you may want to think about this question. Studies have shown that loss of sleep increases the intensity of IBS symptoms. In fact, the amount of sleep you get affects your mental, emotional, and physical health.

What Happens When You Sleep?

There are five stages of sleep, each with a role in helping you get the physical, mental, and emotional rest and renewal that you need.

Stage 1

The first stage of sleep is a transition period between wakefulness and sleep. It is usually completed in about 10 minutes. This is a period of very light sleep during which you are somewhat aware of your surroundings. Most people awakened during this stage of sleep believe that they have not been asleep.

Stage 2

Stage 2 lasts about 10 to 20 minutes and is considered the beginning of actual sleep. During this stage, you disengage from your environment but if awakened, you will feel alert and aware of your surroundings.

Stages 3 and 4

Stages 3 and 4 are deeper stages of sleep, each with specific brain activity patterns. They are restorative in nature. Stage 4 is vital for growth, physical recuperation, and maintaining the immune system. People who are deprived of stage 4 sleep experience fatigue and muscle aches. Because stages 3 and 4 are very deep stages of sleep, if you are awakened during either one, you will feel groggy and disoriented.

REM Sleep

After about 30 to 40 minutes of stage 4 sleep, you generally return to stage 3 and then stage 2 sleep. Generally, you do not return to stage 1 unless you wake up. Following stage 2, you enter rapid eye movement (REM) sleep. This stage of sleep lasts between 1 and 10 minutes and is marked by dreams and rapid eye movement. REM sleep is required for memory storage, retention, organization, and reorganization. Neurotransmitters, which are essential for learning and a sense of emotional well-being, are replenished during this stage of sleep. People who are deprived of REM sleep experience irritability, moodiness, and memory problems.

After the first period of REM sleep, you generally cycle through stage 2, stage 3, and stage 4 sleep 1 or 2 more times before you return again to another period of REM sleep. During eight continuous hours of sleep, you will usually have 4 to 6 episodes of REM sleep, with each episode getting longer as the night progresses. The majority of your REM sleep occurs at the end of the night. It is important to get several continuous hours of sleep to get enough REM sleep.

Insomnia

Insomnia is poor or inadequate sleep characterized by one or more of the following:

- difficulty falling asleep
- difficulty staying asleep
- waking up too early in the morning
- sleep that is not refreshing

Everyone has difficulty sleeping at times. Having a cup of coffee with your dessert at dinner, worrying about your finances, or even watching the evening news can at times cause you to have difficulty falling asleep or staying asleep through the night. If you begin to have difficulty sleeping, it is important that you take some steps to deal with the problem quickly so that occasional insomnia does not become a chronic, ongoing problem. Remain aware of your thought patterns if you have difficulty sleeping. Worrying about your sleep or lying in bed fuming about how tired you will be tomorrow will significantly decrease your chances of sleeping. A healthier choice is to turn the clock away from the bed and practice your favorite relaxation exercise, focusing on how pleasant it feels to relax.

Most people with IBS find that lack of sleep, even for a short period, increases the intensity or severity of their symptoms. One aspect of mastering your IBS symptoms is practicing simple ways of promoting sleep. It's not just about bedtime. Good sleep habits involve your health, lifestyle, and environment, all of which affect how well you sleep. Read the following suggestions and think about any changes that might help improve or ensure your sleep.

Good Sleep Habits

- Go to bed and get up at the same time each day.
- Don't sleep in on weekends or holidays.
- Avoid consuming caffeine for 4 to 6 hours before you go to bed. This includes coffee, tea, colas, or chocolate. Some medications, such as preparations that treat cold symptoms, also contain caffeine.
- Avoid using nicotine near bedtime and if you wake up in the night. Nicotine, like caffeine, is a stimulant that can keep you awake.
- Avoid using alcohol to help you relax or fall asleep. Although alcohol can make you sleepy, it interferes with your REM sleep.
- Take prescribed medications at the correct time of day. Some medicines cause difficulty sleeping. Discuss this with your health care provider.
- Avoid heavy meals in the late evening.
- Do not go to bed hungry. A light snack before bedtime may help you sleep.
- Avoid vigorous exercise 3 to 4 hours before bedtime; this may interfere with your sleep. Regular exercise during the day or in the late afternoon will help you sleep.
- Minimize light, noise, and extreme temperatures while you are sleeping. Some people find it helpful to turn on a fan or use a white noise machine at night to drown out noises that might keep them awake.
- Do something relaxing before you go to bed. Watching the news, engaging in tense conversations, or reading mysteries or the newspaper at bedtime can cause stress or anxiety that may make it difficult to fall or stay asleep.
- Pay attention to your thinking as you are lying in bed. You have identified problematic thought patterns that are most common for you. Be alert for these and change them to more accurate, calming thoughts as soon as possible
- If you are worried that you'll forget something, get up and write it down. Then tell yourself to not worry about it until the morning.
- Use the relaxation exercises that you find most helpful. Try the autogenic exercise that is explained in Chapter 8.
- If you are unable to sleep, get up and go to another room. Do something relaxing such as reading or a gentle stretching exercise until you feel tired. Then go back to bed.
- Don't keep looking at the clock through the night, worrying that you will be tired in the morning. This will cause you to feel anxious and keep you awake. Some people find it helpful to turn the clock around so that the face is not visible.

As Dan learned more about sleep, he was able to set up a plan that significantly improved his sleep and decreased his IBS symptoms. First, he decided to cut down on his intake of caffeine. The constant fatigue had led to an increase in his coffee and cola consumption. His goals were to limit his caffeine to a maximum of one 8- or 12-oz. cup of coffee in the morning and one 12-oz. cola in the early afternoon and to get to bed at 11:00 p.m. each evening and get up at 6:30 a.m. each morning. Dan created a "buffer zone" around his bedtime. At 10:00 p.m., his plan was to begin to wind down. The last hour of the day was spent relaxing in the hot tub, talking to his wife, reading a calming magazine or book, or doing a relaxation exercise. This worked for many days, but life had a way of interfering. Some nights, he would see an upsetting story on the news; some nights, his wife said she needed to discuss something that could not wait. But on nights when he could follow his plan, this buffer zone became his favorite time of the day. Darker curtains and a fan in his room helped to create an environment conducive to sleep. Finally, he turned the clock away from his bed. If he wakes up during the night now, he uses his breathing exercises and focuses on savoring the sense of feeling relaxed.

Now that you have reviewed the good sleep habit suggestions, list the ones that you can use the next time you have trouble sleeping.

1.

2.

3.

4.

Sleep Diary

If you have trouble sleeping, use the suggestions that you have chosen for several nights. Keep track of your sleep in the Sleep Diary; you will find extra copies in the Appendix.

Recognizing the importance of managing his brief episode of insomnia, Dan decided to monitor his sleep with the Sleep Diary for a week to see if his plan was helping to improve his sleep.

Dan's Sleep Diary

Day number and date	Last night I went to bed at:	Last night I fell asleep at:	Number of times I woke up during the night	I got up at:	Number of hours that I slept	When I awoke, I felt: (circle one)	My sleep was disturbed by: (mental, emotional, physical, or environmental factors)
Day 1 7/8 date	11:00 am/(pm)	11:15 am/(pm)	3 # of times	6:00 (am)/pm	6 3/4 hours	Refreshed Somewhat refreshed (Fatigued)	*Emotional–a little worry about sleep*
Day 2 7/9 date	11:00 am/(pm)	11:20 am/(pm)	1 # of times	6:15 (am)/pm	7 hours	Refreshed (Somewhat refreshed) Fatigued	*Nothing*
Day 3 7/10 date	11:00 am/(pm)	11:15 am/(pm)	2 # of times	7:00 (am)/pm	7.5 hours	(Refreshed) Somewhat refreshed Fatigued	*Worry about sleep*
Day 4 7/11 date	11:00 am/(pm)	11:15 am/(pm)	1 # of times	6:30 (am)/pm	7 hours	refreshed (Somewhat refreshed) Fatigued	*Noisy garbage truck*
Day 5 7/12 date	11:00 am/(pm)	11:15 am/(pm)	0 # of times	6:15 (am)/pm	7 hours	Refreshed (Somewhat refreshed) Fatigued	*Nothing*
Day 6 7/13 date	11:10 am/(pm)	11:25 am/(pm)	0 # of times	6:30 (am)/pm	7 hours	Refreshed (Somewhat refreshed) Fatigued	*Nothing*
Day 7 7/14 date	11:00 am/(pm)	11:15 am/(pm)	0 # of times	6:15 (am)/pm	7 hours	Refreshed (Somewhat refreshed) Fatigued	*Nothing*

Dan found that the Sleep Diary was a helpful way to remember how he slept. On most nights, he was able to see that less than 7 hours of sleep a night didn't leave him feeling rested in the morning. Seven and a half hours left him feeling refreshed and ready to face the day. Keeping the Sleep Diary also helped him to avoid worry about his sleep. He could see that his sleep was improving, and most nights he got enough sleep to feel at least "somewhat refreshed" in the morning.

 Sleep Diary

Day number and date	Last night I went to bed at:	Last night I fell asleep at:	Number of times I woke up during the night	I got up at:	Number of hours that I slept	When I awoke, I felt: (circle one)	My sleep was disturbed by: (mental, emotional, physical, or environmental factors)
Day 1 date	am/pm	am/pm	# of times	am/pm	hours	Refreshed Somewhat refreshed Fatigued	
Day 2 date	am/pm	am/pm	# of times	am/pm	hours	Refreshed Somewhat refreshed Fatigued	
Day 3 date	am/pm	am/pm	# of times	am/pm	hours	Refreshed Somewhat refreshed Fatigued	
Day 4 date	am/pm	am/pm	# of times	am/pm	hours	Refreshed Somewhat refreshed Fatigued	
Day 5 date	am/pm	am/pm	# of times	am/pm	hours	Refreshed Somewhat refreshed Fatigued	
Day 6 date	am/pm	am/pm	# of times	am/pm	hours	Refreshed Somewhat refreshed Fatigued	
Day 7 date	am/pm	am/pm	# of times	am/pm	hours	Refreshed Somewhat refreshed Fatigued	

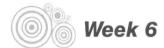 *Week 6*

Skills to Build

Relaxation

Continue the quieting response or abdominal breathing exercise 6 to 8 times a day.

Practice the visualization exercise 1 to 2 times this week.

Choose 1 or 2 good sleep habit suggestions to try if you have trouble sleeping.

Planning

Use the Pain Management Plan to develop your plan to manage pain.

Self-Awareness

Complete the Keeping Track form each day.

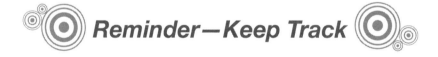

Mini-Relaxation Exercises

> ### IN THIS CHAPTER
>
> Learn short relaxation exercises that you can do throughout your day to help you stay relaxed.
>
> ### QUICK FACTS
>
> You can use a short autogenic exercise or a short progressive muscle relaxation exercise multiple times during your day.

Relaxation Anytime, Anywhere

Mini-relaxation exercises can be a great way to relax during the day. They are short exercises that can be done in a variety of places that you might be throughout your day. When done frequently during the day, the exercises can help you to remain relaxed and calm in spite of your environment. The quieting response and abdominal breathing exercise are examples of mini-relaxation exercises.

You have also learned to do longer relaxation exercises such as active progressive muscle relaxation, passive progressive muscle relaxation, visualization, and autogenic exercises. Now that you are skilled at these exercises, you will be able to do shortened versions of them with only a little practice.

The first mini-relaxation exercise is an abbreviated active progressive muscle relaxation exercise. In this exercise, you tighten and then relax several muscle groups at one time. Read through the instructions below, and then try the exercise. Do not worry about getting it exactly right. The goal is to relax.

Abbreviated Active Progressive Muscle Relaxation

- Tighten the muscles in both arms and hands, and focus on the tension that you experience. Hold the tension for 5 seconds. Now relax your muscles and focus on the feeling of relaxation in your arms and hands.
- Tighten the muscles in your head, neck, and shoulders. Hold the tension for 5 seconds, focusing on the tension that you feel. Relax and enjoy the sense of relaxation in your head, neck, and shoulders.
- Take a deep breath and hold it. Now tighten the muscles in your chest, back, and abdomen. Hold the tension for 5 seconds. Slowly exhale and relax, focusing on the feeling of relaxation in that area.
- Tighten the muscles in your hips, buttocks, thighs, calves, and feet. Hold the tension for 5 seconds. Relax the tension, and focus on the overall state of relaxation that you feel.

Wave of Relaxation

- Take a slow, deep breath.
- Imagine that a wave of relaxation starts at your head and travels down through your body.
- Let the sensation of warmth and heaviness relax your entire body as the wave passes from your head and neck through your arms, trunk, legs, feet, and flows out of your toes.
- Spend a minute savoring the sensation of relaxation.
- Take another slow, deep breath and then return to your normal activities.

Remember that the progression of the exercise is:

> Tighten muscle group →
> Focus → Relax muscle
> group → Focus

The next exercise uses your passive relaxation, visualization, and autogenic skills. With practice, you will learn to feel a warm "wave of relaxation" traveling down through your body. Some people find it helpful to imagine that there is a soft, warm light shining on the tops of their heads and moving down toward their feet. As the wave passes through your body, you'll feel a warming sensation. Other people find that it is helpful to imagine that someone is pouring warm, soothing, fragrant oil over their bodies from head to toe. Try the exercise and see which vision you prefer.

Molly occasionally splurged on a massage to relax. The warm, pleasant-smelling massage oil was a helpful visualization for her. The warmth and smell of the oil reminded her of the relaxation she experienced after a massage.

Beth imagined a soft, warm light inside of her. It warmed and relaxed her from the inside out. The idea of inner warmth helped her to relax more deeply than a source of warmth outside of her body.

James found it easier to imagine that the sun was warming him. He could easily imagine and feel the warmth of the sun on his body.

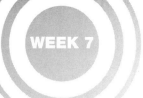
Stretching Your Comfort Zone

> ### IN THIS CHAPTER
>
> Learn from the suggestions of others with IBS about how to make eating out and traveling enjoyable experiences.
>
> ### QUICK FACTS
>
> Many people with IBS dread eating out and traveling because these experiences aggravate their IBS symptoms.
>
> You can adapt the strategies you have already learned to help you deal with changes in food, water, eating habits, sleep patterns, and daily routine.
>
> Remember that food storage and preparation away from home can sometimes cause "safe" foods to become trigger foods.

Eating Out

Mara's day at work had been crazy. She had worked late and missed the bus she had planned to take but was now on her way downtown to meet her husband and some of his coworkers for dinner. Reaching into her purse for the granola bar that she kept there, she remembered that she ate it for lunch yesterday. "Oh well, we'll have dinner soon." Mara hopped off the bus and walked the few blocks to the restaurant, trying to remember when she ate last. No wonder she was so hungry—she had grabbed an apple for lunch at about noon. That was 7 hours ago! She knew that she needed to eat more often to manage her IBS symptoms.

Walking into the restaurant, she saw her husband and his coworkers having drinks at the bar. She felt her stomach tighten a little as she walked over to the group. They welcomed her warmly and told her that their table would be ready at 7:30. Mara ordered a glass of wine and settled into the seat next to her husband. At about 7:40 they were seated at their table. The laughter and conversation continued, but all Mara could think about was that she was starving. After a few minutes, the waiter came to their table. The menu was full of wonderful choices. Mara decided on a Caesar salad, grilled salmon, garlic mashed potatoes, and broccoli. By 8:15, their salads were served. The Caesar salad was large and delicious; Mara ate it all. Feeling better, she was able to relax. The salmon arrived soon after the salad and Mara started her dinner. Without really thinking, Mara finished her entire dinner. Then, bloating and abdominal discomfort replaced the hunger pains she had felt earlier. Her skirt felt tight, and she began to worry about how long they might have to stay.

Mara's pain and bloating had increased by the time they left the restaurant. The trip home was miserable. Soon after they got home, the urgency and diarrhea started. Mara spent most of the night in pain.

Have you found that eating out is a difficult experience? By using all of the skills that you have been practicing, you can make eating away from home a more relaxed and pleasurable experience. The preparation for an enjoyable meal starts before you reach the restaurant.

Changing Your Thoughts

Begin by paying attention to any problematic thought patterns you have. Watch for thoughts like these:

> "I always get sick when I eat out."
> "It isn't fair that I always have to be so careful about what I eat."
> "I think I'll just stay home so I don't have to worry about how I'll feel afterward."

As you recognize these thoughts, you can replace them with more positive, accurate thoughts, such as:

> "It's too bad that I have IBS, but there are things I can do to manage my symptoms."
> "I am much more in control than I used to be."
> "If I relax and don't worry so much about eating out, I'm more likely to enjoy the meal."

Calming your mind can also help you prepare for a meal away from home. Remind yourself to "relax." Try repeating the word "relax" or another calming word to yourself when you begin to feel anxious or worried. Changing your focus to something other than your worries or concerns will help you relax. Accurate statements such as, "I will feel better when I relax," will also help you feel calmer.

Relaxation Exercises

Many of our study participants find it helpful to use their favorite relaxation exercise before they go out to eat. Increasing the number of times you do the quieting response or abdominal breathing prior to your meal out can be an effective way of relaxing. Plan ahead so that you can take 10 or 15 minutes to do a longer relaxation exercise before you leave home.

Diet

Before you go out for a meal, think about what you would like to eat. Do you want to just go for whatever looks good on the menu and possibly suffer the consequences later? Or do you want to carefully review the menu and choose foods that are less likely to lead to an increase in your IBS symptoms? Either choice is fine. Sometimes it is nice to have whatever you want to eat, and other times it is more comfortable to choose foods that probably won't lead to IBS symptoms.

By this time, you have learned a great deal about your body and managing your symptoms. Your symptoms do not control you. If you choose to have foods that sound good but may increase your symptoms, you might feel uncomfortable but it will not damage your body, and you have skills to minimize the symptoms if you need them. Here are several suggestions that you might find useful.

- Eat before you go. Have a small low-fat snack so that you are not hungry when you arrive.
- Appetizers are often high in fat. Only have a bite or two, or choose low-fat appetizers such as bread, breadsticks, pretzels, or a fruit plate.
- Avoid or limit alcohol if you have difficulty tolerating it.
- Some people find that they feel better if they do not have a salad before dinner. If you choose to have a salad, ask for the dressing on the side and try eating your salad with your meal instead of before.

Many people report that Caesar salads cause more IBS symptoms than simple green salads. Other people find that iceberg lettuce is more difficult to tolerate than other types of lettuce.

- Choose menu items that are low in fat. Lean meats such as chicken, fish, or lean cuts of pork are good choices.

- Don't hesitate to ask how foods are prepared. Foods that are broiled, baked, barbecued, braised, roasted, steamed, stewed, stir-fried, or poached usually are low in fat. Avoid deep-fried foods. Many people are surprised to learn that Chinese food is often quite high in fat. You can ask that less oil be used in cooking. Thai food, however, seems to be tolerated by many of our study participants if it is not overly spicy.

- Eat small portions of food. Take part of your meal home or just leave it on your plate. Think about sharing an entree with a family member or a friend. It is also an option when you order to ask for half the food to be served on your plate and half of the food to be put in a take-out container for you to take home.

- If you decide to have dessert, choose something that is low in fat, such as fruit, angel food cake, frozen yogurt, or sorbet. You may enjoy ordering a fruit-based dessert, such as apple crisp or berry pie, and eating just the fruit.

- Wear loose-fitting clothes. Avoid tight-fitting jeans, skirts, or panty hose. Loosen your belt if possible.

- Some restaurants print the calories contained in each item on their menu. In some places, you have to ask for this menu; in other places, it is on every menu. Take advantage of this information. Items that have fewer calories often have less fat. You may find that some salads have more calories than a grilled chicken sandwich.

- Eat slowly.

- Eat in a quiet, relaxed setting when you have the opportunity. Use the quieting response to help you stay relaxed while you are eating.

- When you finish your meal, get up and move around. Just a short walk to the restroom can be enough movement to help you feel relaxed and comfortable.

- If you are having a meal at someone's home, offer to bring a food that you enjoy. Take something that is low in fat and that you know you will tolerate.

Having IBS is not uncommon. Consider telling your host or hostess about your dietary needs if you are having a meal in someone's home. If you are going out to a restaurant with friends, sharing your dietary needs will allow you to choose a restaurant that everyone will enjoy.

Throughout the world, sharing a meal is the way people establish and nurture relationships with others. Despite your IBS, eating out can be an enjoyable experience. Try some of the suggestions given above and decide which ones work for you. Try using some strategies from each category, to increase your chances for success.

Travel

Lying on the cold, hard bathroom floor of her hotel room, Erika curled up into a ball waiting for the cramping and pain to subside. Her symptoms were most severe when she traveled. She dreaded these business trips. The stress of making presentations and not knowing when the pain would start seemed like more than she could bear. She had tried only sipping liquids for the entire trip; another time, she had tried eating only soda crackers and ice chips. Nothing seemed to help.

Travel poses some of the same challenges as eating out, and a few additional ones. Making use of all of the strategies you have learned will be helpful when you travel.

If you are on vacation, do your best to leave the concerns of home and work behind. As you begin to relax, you may find that your symptoms decrease and you are able to tolerate foods that aggravate symptoms when you are at home.

If you are on a business trip, you can decrease your anxiety by planning ahead. Find out what restaurants are near your hotel, what your schedule will be, whether there is an exercise facility nearby, and if you'll have a refrigerator in your room. If there is a required banquet, see if you can request a low-fat meal. Use the strategies that are effective at home to make travel more enjoyable.

Changing Your Thoughts

Pay attention to your thought patterns as you are planning the trip. Are you worrying? Do you expect to be miserable? Are you remembering past negative experiences and assuming that this trip will be the same? Identify your problem thoughts and work to change what you are thinking. The sooner you begin this process, the less stressed you will feel.

Many of our study participants feel anxious about flying. They begin worrying days ahead of time. Their symptoms increase when they reach the airport, and this increases their anxiety. It becomes a vicious cycle—anxiety increasing symptoms, symptoms increasing anxiety—and the cycle goes on, making the trip very uncomfortable. Pay careful attention to your thoughts about flying. Use the Problem Solving worksheet to think about alternatives to worrying about flying.

Relaxation

Use the relaxation exercises that you find the most effective. While you are traveling, use a mini-relaxation exercise such as abdominal breathing, the quieting response, and any other kind of relaxation that works well for you. Try deep breathing while you are driving or on the plane to your destination, so you can arrive much more relaxed. Use the longer relaxation exercises on a regular basis throughout the trip.

Take time to move around while you are traveling. Get in the habit of taking short, frequent walks, using the stairs instead of the escalator, and standing up to stretch during plane or train trips. Having a comfortable, broken-in pair of walking shoes will encourage you to do this. If you are on a road trip, stop often and get out of the car to take a short walk.

Plan relaxing activities to enjoy while you are on your trip. Find out about the area you are visiting before you leave home. Identify activities that you enjoy and work them into your schedule. Be as active as possible when you travel. This might mean playing tennis, swimming, hiking, or parking a short distance from your destination and walking the final block or two.

Diet

When you travel, you have less control over your food than when you are at home. Try to maintain as many of your usual eating strategies as you can. For example, continue eating every 3 to 4 hours, avoid high-fat meals, get an adequate amount of fiber in your diet, and drink plenty of water. It is not always easy to maintain these habits. Here are a few suggestions that will help you.

- Keep healthy snacks in your car, pocket, travel bag, or purse.
- Avoid drinking sodas. Drink juice and water. Some people prefer to drink bottled water when they are traveling.
- Keep track of your fluid intake. Drink about 64 ounces of water or juice a day.

- Take fruit with you. It is often difficult to get enough fruit when you are eating out. Keep fresh fruit handy for snacks. If you tolerate dried fruit, carry some raisins, apples, cherries, or peaches.
- If you tend to get constipated when you travel, pack a fiber supplement such as FiberCon, Citrucel, or Metamucil. Remember to drink at least 8 ounces of water with each dose of these supplements.
- Avoid fast food restaurants whenever possible. Lower fat options at fast food restaurants include a plain hamburger, a grilled chicken sandwich without mayonnaise, an egg sandwich without bacon or sausage, a salad with a low-fat dressing, and frozen yogurt.
- Try to prepare some of your own meals. Stop at a grocery store to buy some healthy, easy-to-prepare foods. Some foods that you can prepare in a hotel room with a refrigerator and microwave include instant oatmeal packets with fruit, cold whole-grain cereal, instant soups, sandwiches, pull-top canned tuna with whole-grain crackers, fresh fruits and vegetables, and low-fat frozen entrées. Having your own food with you gives you more control over your eating schedule as well as your fat and fiber intake.

As Erika learned more about the struggles of managing IBS during travel, she was able to develop a plan that worked for her. She typically noticed that the pain began before she even got on the plane. Just the worry about being stuck in her seat when she needed to use the restroom seemed to lead to pain. Then there was the worry about actually using the restrooms on the plane; that increased her anxiety even more. With new understanding of the impact of her thoughts on her feelings and symptoms, Erika worked to change her thinking. She changed her worried thoughts to

> "I have a seat on the aisle. It will be easy to get to the restroom when I need to."
> "I will use the restroom at the airport before I get on the plane and then I will focus on doing a relaxation exercise and reading a magazine when I get on the plane."

Relaxation now plays an important role in the management of her symptoms when she travels. Erika closes her eyes and begins doing an autogenic exercise the minute she is settled on the plane. She begins each day with several minutes of abdominal breathing before she even gets out of bed. The quieting response is a routine part of her day, and she spends some time each afternoon doing a passive progressive muscle relaxation exercise. Erika generally eats breakfast in her hotel room and then goes out for a walk before her business meetings begin.

Erika tried several fiber supplements before she found one that she tolerated well. Now she never travels without it. She has learned to pack high-fiber snack bars in her suitcase and carry-on bag. When she arrives at her destination, she makes a trip to the grocery store to purchase oatmeal and fresh berries for breakfast; a high-fiber, low-fat cereal, nuts, and a small bag of M&Ms to make a healthy high-fiber trail mix for snacking; some fresh fruit; and one or two frozen low-fat entrées that she can microwave for an occasional dinner. On some trips, she purchases bottled water because the water in various parts of the country seems to aggravate her IBS symptoms.

Erika travels frequently. It took a while for her to get her plan refined to meet her needs. But changing her thoughts, staying relaxed, increasing her fiber and fluid intake, and getting regular exercise now allow her to travel confidently and comfortably. She seldom suffers with her IBS symptoms when she travels, and when she does experience symptoms, they are mild and easily managed.

Travel can be a relaxing, enjoyable experience, even if you have IBS. Experiment with some of the suggestions in this chapter and identify the ones that are most effective for you.

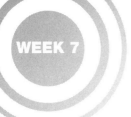

Physical Intimacy

IN THIS CHAPTER

Consider how IBS symptoms affect your approach to sex and learn changes you can make to lessen the impact of IBS.

QUICK FACTS

Many people with IBS report decreased interest in physical intimacy or lessening of satisfaction with sex.

Pain and embarrassment are the two biggest issues.

You can apply the skills you are using to lessen your symptoms to help make sexual experiences more comfortable and more enjoyable.

Sex and IBS

Many people with IBS, in fact more than 40%, report a decrease in sexual interest, functioning, and satisfaction. These sexual changes include a decrease in sexual drive, IBS symptoms directly preventing intercourse, an increase in sexual problems when IBS symptoms increase, and pain during intercourse. Both men and women experience these symptoms. A decrease in sexual drive is reported almost equally by men and women, but pain during intercourse is more common among women. Other symptoms such as abdominal pain, gas, and bloating can also make intercourse less pleasurable.

Embarrassment and worry related to IBS symptoms can have a profound effect on sexual experiences. Topics such as diarrhea, constipation, gas, bloating, and cramping are not easy to talk about. Although these are common body functions, people with IBS are often overly self-conscious when they occur. The shame and embarrassment associated with these symptoms may cause people with IBS to feel uncomfortable with physical intimacy and to avoid closeness with others.

Stress and Sex

Some sexual problems are directly related to an inability to relax. It is hard to relax if you are worried or your body is tense. Expressing your anxiety to your partner may help you relax. You may find that your partner is not nearly as bothered by IBS symptoms as you imagine. Let your partner know what hurts and what helps you to relax, so you both can feel more successful in expressing love for each other.

Take time to relax, calming your body and your mind before sexual experiences. Your ability to experience and enjoy your sexuality will increase as your tension levels decrease. Intercourse itself can be a healthy source of relaxation, providing a deep sense of pleasure and release from the tension of the day.

Communication with Your Partner

Communication between you and your partner is one key to improving intimacy and sexual relations. For a variety of reasons, it can be difficult to talk seriously about sex. Your beliefs, past experiences, and thought patterns all influence how easy (or difficult) it is for you to talk openly with your partner about your sexual needs and feelings.

Gretchen told her boyfriend Brett about her IBS shortly after she had a sense that this might be a lasting relationship. That first conversation was not an easy one, but she chose a relaxed, low-key afternoon when they were talking about their feelings for one another. She brought up the topic of "things that might affect our relationship." They discussed their past relationships, experiences, and fears. Then she casually mentioned that she had IBS, that it affected her life, and that it would probably affect their relationship in some ways. She didn't go into great detail that day, but she did say that she suffered with abdominal pain, cramping, and urgency. She told Brett that her symptoms were affected by stress and that a healthy lifestyle was her way of effectively managing the symptoms.

That initial conversation was the foundation for further discussion. From there, she was able to identify for Brett specific ways that she managed her symptoms. Brett learned that healthy thought patterns, eating every 3 to 4 hours, staying relaxed, and getting regular exercise and enough sleep helped Gretchen manage her IBS symptoms. Several months later, it seemed natural to talk about strategies that would make their sexual life comfortable and enjoyable. Gretchen included Brett in the problem-solving process, and together they came up with a relaxing and enjoyable plan that works well for them. They have discovered that soft music, back rubs, and taking baths together helps them both relax and extends and increases sexual pleasure for both of them. Gretchen finds it helpful to plan ahead so that she can avoid eating for several hours before intercourse, although spontaneity has a role in their sexual experiences also.

Gretchen and Brett have been married for three years now and are expecting their first child. They would both agree that Gretchen's IBS symptoms have not stifled their sexual pleasure. Their creative spirits, open communication, commitment to a healthy lifestyle, and willingness to experiment have all contributed to the creation of a unique and delightful sexual relationship.

Give some thought to your own feelings about sex. What interferes with your ability to express yourself to your partner? Keep in mind that sex is a normal, healthy part of loving human relationships. Use your cognitive restructuring skills to change your thoughts about ways of bringing up the topic with your partner. Your partner may also find it difficult to talk about sex. Try planning what you want to say and expressing your thoughts in a relaxed environment. As you talk about your sexual concerns, discuss your feelings about your IBS symptoms. When you become more comfortable talking about your body and sexuality, your partner will probably relax as well. Open communication helps strengthen loving relationships.

Suggestions for Success

You have learned many skills that will be of use as you work through sexual struggles. Table 8 provides cognitive, relaxation, dietary, and problem-solving strategies to help make sexual experiences more comfortable and more enjoyable.

Crystal and Zac have been married for two years. Crystal has had IBS since her early teen years. She suffers from abdominal pain, gas, bloating, and diarrhea. Over the past several months, her symptoms have increased in both frequency and intensity. With this increase, Crystal has found that intercourse is painful and unpleasant. Unintentionally, she has pulled away from Zac, not wanting to be touched, kissed, or to even go to bed at the same time. They both have felt the tension increasing.

Chatting with a close friend who also has IBS, Crystal mentioned the struggle she and Zac have been experiencing. Having experienced a similar struggle, Crystal's friend encouraged her to talk with her husband about her

Table 8. Strategies for Successful Physical Intimacy

Strategy	Suggestions
Cognitive Strategies	• Be aware of your thoughts about sexual experiences. Avoid negative thoughts that lead to feelings of fear, dread, or apprehension. • Identify and challenge beliefs that lead to feelings of shame and embarrassment. • Work with your partner to create a sense of anticipation before sexual activity. • Relax your expectations. Remember that intercourse does not always need to be included in your time of intimacy. Closeness, touch, and creative communication can be fulfilling.
Dietary Strategies	• Avoid trigger foods before sexual activity. • Experiment with small meals or no meals before sexual activity.
Relaxation Strategies	• Be consistent with your relaxation exercises during the day. Use the quieting response, abdominal breathing, or another mini-relaxation exercise frequently. • Try a longer relaxation exercise prior to sexual activity. • Take a warm bath or shower to relax. • Ask your partner to give you a back rub or body massage to help you relax and get into a romantic mood. • Purchase a CD of relaxation exercises and listen to it with your partner on occasion and before sexual activity. • Use foreplay as a way to relax further.
Problem-Solving Strategies	• Plan ahead; make a date for a time of intimacy. • Experiment with a variety of times for sexual activity—different times of day or before or after meals. • Identify times when your symptoms are minimal or absent. Plan sexual activity during these times. • Be creative with positions. Try positions that put light or no pressure on your abdomen. Try lying on your side while cuddling. • Get up and use the bathroom between foreplay and intercourse. • Purchase a book on sex and read it with your partner. Talk about creative ideas that might add new sparkle and dimension to your relationship.

feelings. Crystal and Zac have never talked about sex. Crystal didn't even know how to bring it up. After some thought, Crystal decided that she would be able to bring up the topic of the tension between them. Then she might be able to tell Zac that her IBS symptoms have increased recently and that she thought the pain was contributing to the tension they were both feeling. She would tell him that the pain was the worst at night and that sometimes she didn't even want to be touched. Maybe he would understand that the problem really hasn't been him, but that sex is very painful for her when her IBS symptoms are bad.

Gathering all of her courage, Crystal brought up the topic of the tension they were feeling. After a few minutes, they were able to relax and discuss the impact of Crystal's symptoms. Zac was relieved to understand the issue. They talked for a long time that night and came up with a plan. Crystal made appointments with her primary care doctor and her gynecologist. She began to develop a plan that would help her get her symptoms under control. Although, it took a while to feel better, Zac was able to be patient and encouraging because he understood the problem.

When Crystal began feeling better, she was surprised to find that she still dreaded the thought of sex. She was afraid that it would cause the symptoms to increase once again. Crystal and Zac were comfortable talking now, and she was able to share her fears with him. Recognizing that her fears were now the root of the problem, Crystal began working on changing them. She spent a few minutes each day journaling about her thoughts and pushing herself to entertain new thoughts that would free her from her fears. Fairly quickly she was able to identify healthy, accurate thoughts.

"I won't know if sex is painful until we try it again."
"It wasn't painful before my symptoms got worse."
"Zac will help me relax if I ask him."

Crystal did ask him. Together they worked on a slow, gentle pace that helped her relax, new positions that didn't put pressure on her abdomen, and talking about sex before they began so that Crystal knew what to expect. Soon Crystal's confidence began to build and her fears faded. The process that Crystal and Zac worked through took some time, but it has also taught them skills that will be a benefit for years to come.

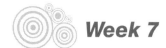 *Week 7*

Skills to Build

Relaxation

Continue the quieting response or abdominal breathing exercise 6 to 8 times a day.

Practice the mini-relaxation exercises (abbreviated active progressive muscle relaxation exercise and wave of relaxation) 1 to 2 times each this week.

Thoughts

Identify 1 or 2 strategies for eating out or travel that may be of help to you in the future.

Identify 1 or 2 strategies that may be of help to you if your IBS affects your sexual experiences in a negative manner.

Think back over all of the strategies that you have tried over the past few weeks. Identify the ones that have been most effective for you.

Self-Awareness

Complete the Keeping Track form each day.

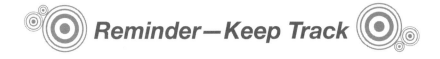 *Reminder—Keep Track*

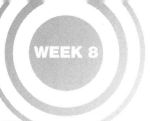

A Comprehensive Plan

IN THIS CHAPTER

Create an overall plan for how you will manage your IBS symptoms.

QUICK FACTS

You have learned many ways to manage your IBS symptoms over the past 7 weeks. It's time to look ahead.

Your comprehensive plan includes those symptom control strategies that you have found most helpful in managing your symptoms.

Putting It All Together

You have worked in the past 7 weeks toward the goal of building skills to self-manage your IBS symptoms. Have you become more aware of what causes your IBS to "flare up"? Have you learned ways to control your symptoms? Then it's time to write a comprehensive plan to continue the progress you've made.

By now, you are aware of the stressors in your life that are connected to your IBS symptoms. You understand how to problem solve to determine what to do next. However, at times of stress (such as when IBS flares up), it is harder to stop and think rationally. This is why planning ahead is important.

Make a written plan that includes how you will respond to specific stressors. Not only does this plan give you a quick reference to use in an emergency, it also forces you to think carefully about how you want to organize your daily life in the future so that you continue minimizing the discomfort and inconvenience of IBS. The plan represents a commitment to yourself that you will manage your symptoms in a consistent manner.

Your plan will give you many ways to manage your IBS symptoms. You have had a chance to practice many strategies and make the most effective ones a part of your daily routine. Managing IBS is an ongoing process that takes time, work, practice, and patience. Some changes you have made involve changing a lifetime of beliefs and behaviors. That's not an easy task!

When you are feeling better, it's easy to go back to old habits. But, wouldn't you rather continue to feel better and better? Practice the skills and concepts you've learned in this book and follow your written plan so that your IBS symptoms play the smallest role possible in your life.

What to Put in Your Plan

Your goal is to maintain and keep improving your skills in managing your IBS. You will fulfill this goal by designing a strategy that focuses on the following behaviors:

- Relaxation techniques: Continue using those that were most effective for you. Relaxation can include more than just relaxation exercises. Think about additional ways that you relax; for example, exercise, reading, talking with friends, warm baths, massage, and hobbies. Relaxation exercises help you achieve deep relaxation, and activities provide a sense of balance and a pace of life that helps you deal with the stresses you face.
- Healthy thoughts: Continue identifying and changing problematic ways of thinking; challenge false beliefs. Which problematic thought patterns do you need to continue to focus on? How have you used problem-solving skills?
- Dietary strategies: Focus on eating small, frequent, well-balanced meals; taking recommended vitamins and minerals; avoiding or limiting specific trigger foods; and getting adequate amounts of fiber and fluids.

How have you used each of these behaviors for overall symptom management in the past weeks? How have you used them to help you with specific challenges such as eating out, travel, managing your pain, and sleeping well?

The best plan is as specific as you can make it. Telling yourself that you need to "do a better job dealing with stress" or "relax more" is vague and won't guide you to your goal. Think about the strategies that effectively helped you to relax.

Include everything that you want to continue doing to manage your IBS symptoms. If your symptoms increase at a later point, you can come back to this plan and get right back on track.

Cheryl has identified several strategies that allow her to eat out with minimal or no symptoms. She wants to include them in her plan.

Diet
- Eat oatmeal and fruit for breakfast before going to work.
- Include some fiber in every meal or snack.
- Avoid coffee on an empty stomach. Drink herbal tea if my symptoms are a problem.
- Limit cruciferous vegetables to one a day.
- Eat a small low-fat snack before going out to dinner.
- Avoid trigger foods when eating out.
- Take at least half of my meal home when I eat out.

Relaxation
- Take 5 to 10 slow abdominal breaths 3 to 4 times a day: when I first wake up and am still in bed, midmorning, right before I leave work for the day or begin to prepare dinner, and when I get into bed.
- Spend 15 minutes doing active progressive muscle relaxation or visualization before I go out for dinner or to meet friends.
- Walk for one mile 3 times a week: Mondays and Wednesdays at noon and Sundays after breakfast.

Thoughts
- Continue to pay attention to perfectionist tendencies. Challenge thoughts that say "only perfect is good enough." Remind myself of the evidence that says "my family and friends prefer me to my accomplishments."
- Be aware of my thoughts before I go out to dinner. Don't worry about how the meal will go. Focus on my competency and relax.

Sarah has benefited from recognizing early signs of pain and intervening quickly. This has been especially helpful during busy times at work. A healthy lifestyle has helped to decrease her pain, and when she occasionally experiences discomfort she is able to intervene quickly.

Diet
- Eat small, frequent meals. Keep snacks in my car and desk drawer.
- Avoid trigger foods prior to work deadlines: coffee, chocolate, ice cream, fast foods, raw veggies.
- Eat about 20 grams of fiber every day.
- Fill my large green sports bottle with water and drink 1 bottle each day.

Relaxation
- Use abdominal breathing every hour at work.
- Scan my body for muscle tension with every meal and snack.
- Keep neck and shoulders relaxed.
- When I begin to get upset, take a few minutes alone to do the wave of relaxation exercise.
- Begin Tuesday night yoga class.

Thoughts
- Be alert for overgeneralization and "should" thinking, especially when I am at work. Replace "I should" with "it would be nice if . . ." Change these thoughts as soon as possible to healthy, accurate thoughts.

Samuel travels often for work. He has discovered that he can minimize his symptoms with a healthy lifestyle. With a few additional steps, he can manage his symptoms when he travels.

Diet
- Eat every 3 to 4 hours; always keep high-fiber snacks at work and in my car.
- Eat 7 to 9 servings of fruits and vegetables each day.
- Avoid trigger foods for 2 to 3 days before travel: red meat, cruciferous vegetables, melon, red wine, and fast foods.
- Increase fiber to at least 30 grams a day when traveling.

Relaxation
- Do quieting response 3 to 4 times each day.
- Get up from my desk and stretch every 1 to 2 hours when I am at work.
- Run 2 to 3 miles 3 to 5 days a week.
- Listen to relaxation exercises when I fly.

Thoughts
- Watch for negative overgeneralization thoughts, especially at work. When I become aware that I'm overgeneralizing, move out of the environment and let myself relax. Change the thought to an accurate one.
- Be aware of my thoughts before I travel. Don't worry about flying. This plan works, and I really can manage my symptoms.

These are some suggestions that worked for our study participants. This is the time to write a plan that will work for you. You can personalize it in a way that will be effective for you. Be sure that your plan is specific, measurable, and realistic. Include everything that you want to do to manage your symptoms effectively.

Exercise: Reflection

Take a few minutes to relax using your favorite relaxation technique. Close your eyes if you wish. Let your mind wander back over the past 7 weeks and your experiences learning and practicing new strategies and skills.

Now, ask yourself:

- How do I feel now?
- How did I feel when I started the program?
- Have my symptoms changed?
- What triggered my symptoms—stress, diet, or problematic thoughts?
- What strategies did I find most helpful?
- How did I make these strategies work for me?
- What part was the easiest?
- What was the hardest thing to do or change?

Take a few slow, deep breaths and enjoy the feeling of relaxation. Then slowly open your eyes. Take a few minutes to write down your thoughts. These notes will provide a record of your progress, accomplishments, and difficulties that you can use to create your plan.

Use the form on page 152 to write your comprehensive plan to manage your IBS symptoms.

A Comprehensive Plan for Managing My IBS Symptoms

1. Diet	
2. Relaxation	
3. Thoughts	

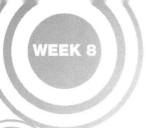

A Plan for the Future

IN THIS CHAPTER

Now that you have a comprehensive plan for controlling your IBS symptoms, learn some strategies for those days that you don't stick to your plan.

QUICK FACTS

Nobody's perfect! Study participants used these behaviors to get back on track:

- Post the plan in a place where you will see it often.
- Post or create reminders.
- Give yourself rewards for successes.
- Tell others about your goals.
- Plan for possible problems.
- Keep a forgiving attitude.
- Be flexible.

Moving Forward

Over the past 8 weeks, you have learned a variety of ways to manage your IBS symptoms. These include making dietary changes, incorporating relaxation exercises and activities into your day, and developing healthier thought patterns. You can use these three skill areas to help you manage your symptoms indefinitely.

Here are the key points we want you to remember:

- Eat nutritious, well-balanced meals.
- Eat regularly, and include healthy snacks between meals.
- Identify and limit foods that trigger symptoms.
- Drink 6 to 8 glasses of water and eat 20 to 35 grams of fiber each day.
- Practice relaxation strategies regularly.
- Be aware of your thought patterns.
- Identify automatic thoughts as they occur.
- Replace problematic thoughts with more accurate, helpful thoughts.
- Use problem-solving skills when you are facing a problem and feel stuck.
- Identify and challenge false beliefs.
- Get plenty of sleep. Most people need 7 to 8 hours of sleep each night.
- Identify strategies that help you manage pain, sleep, eating out, travel, and issues with intimacy.
- Keep a record of what you have done, and reward yourself for doing it.
- Talk with your health care providers about concerns.

Getting Unstuck

Sometimes even the best-laid plans don't work out. The plan may be faulty, or we may find ourselves not following through, not doing as well as we had hoped, or just feeling overwhelmed. It's like the engine has stalled in your car.

If you feel stuck and unable to follow through with your symptoms management plan, start by doing something to relax. This could be a relaxation exercise or doing something you enjoy, like taking a walk, watching a funny movie, or playing with your dog. Once you are a bit more relaxed, go back to thinking about your plan.

What was the category of the problem? Which strategy are you having trouble following through on? It may be too difficult or it just might not be the strategy for you. You might want to set that strategy aside and work on something else for a while. Otherwise, you can keep it and figure out a new way to reach it (change your plan).

Juan was pleased that his IBS symptoms had decreased by the time he finished the study. His plan was more effective than he had expected. He had found it easy to make his relaxation and eating strategies a part of his everyday life. He didn't need to look at his plan or keep track of symptoms or strategies any more.

A few months after he completed the study, Juan was transferred from an evening shift to a day shift. After about a week, his symptoms began to increase. It took a few days for him to realize that, with his new focus on the job change, he had put aside many of his strategies that effectively managed his symptoms. Unknowingly, he had gone from eating small, frequent meals to eating three meals a day, with the largest meal in the evening. Getting up so early made it difficult for him to pack a lunch, so he had been going out to eat each day with coworkers. He also missed his daily morning swim and hadn't replaced it with an alternative form of exercise.

Juan got his comprehensive plan out and began to rethink it. He still needed the same strategies in his life but in a new way. He started packing his lunch and snacks the night before. He still went out to lunch once or twice a week with coworkers, but he ordered soup or half a sandwich instead of a large, higher-fat meal. He struggled to get exercise back into his life. He began stopping at the gym a couple of nights a week and tried to get to the pool twice a week. Each strategy had to be reworked in some way, but he knew where to start and which strategies were the most effective for him. After a few weeks, he was able to get his symptoms under control once again.

If you can't get yourself to do anything at all, try to identify your "top feelings" (the strongest feelings you have) when you think about your IBS or about following your plan. If you feel overwhelmed by it all, you may need to break it down into smaller pieces and not try to do it all at once. If you feel discouraged by continued symptoms, try to identify those strategies that have been most helpful and focus on those.

You may need to give yourself a pep talk to get motivated again. Remind yourself that following your plan or using certain strategies has helped in the past. Not following the plan for a while can be a learning experience. For example, getting off your diet may set off symptoms, although it is not hurting your body. Try to refocus and move on.

Here are some other ways that you can keep on track.

Reminders

Many people fail to follow through on things because they get busy and simply forget. Think of creative ways you can remind yourself of your plans. It may be helpful to post your plan in a place where you see it often, or use sticky notes as reminders on your phone, computer, or mirror.

David set the alarm on his phone to ring at 10:15 a.m., 3:30 p.m., and 7:30 p.m. Each time it goes off, he scans his body for tension and does something to relax. He might get up from his desk and walk to the drinking fountain, do some abdominal breathing, or go for a walk. It is an effective way to have a regular break from the stress of the day.

Amy posted her plan inside a cabinet door in the bathroom. She opens it each morning to get her makeup and reminds herself of the strategies that changed her life.

Rewards

Reward yourself when you complete a task or meet a goal. Rewards can be as simple as a check mark on your to-do list or as special as a dinner out. Recognizing your progress is important because it motivates you to continue. IBS is tough and making these lifestyle changes is difficult. Give yourself credit for all you are accomplishing!

Amber had a difficult time thinking of a reward that didn't defeat her progress. When she thought of rewards, she thought of chocolate, ice cream, lasagna, or Mexican food. She felt as though she was taking one step forward and two steps back. She decided to come up with a list of nonfood rewards and post it on the refrigerator. Her list included getting a pedicure, calling a friend, taking a nap or a warm bath, going for a walk, working on a craft project, buying a new book or magazine, or going to a movie. She continues to add to her list so that she doesn't get bored with the rewards.

Denise found that rewards could be pleasant things that she was already planning on doing. For example, she might decide that, before she watched her favorite TV show, she would take a walk; before she called a friend, she would do a relaxation exercise; before she went shopping, she would use the problem-solving form to think about how to deal with a problem at work. Denise knew that this method gave her day a pleasant rhythm and broke up the stress that might otherwise have triggered her symptoms.

Public Commitment

You may find it helpful to tell a few friends or family members about your plan. Ask for their support. They may also ask you to support them in a plan. You can also find a support group in your area.

Joy thought about asking her husband Tom for support and decided instead to ask her cousin Kristi. She called her cousin and asked her if they could get together or talk by phone every couple of weeks about how she was doing with her comprehensive plan. She told her cousin that she just wanted to know that someone was going to ask her, on a regular basis, how she was doing managing her IBS symptoms. Joy knew that, if for some reason she were to stop the plan, all she would need is some understanding words and a gentle reminder that she feels much better when she is using the strategies on her plan.

Private Commitment

Don't set a goal that you don't believe in, don't understand, or can't feel committed to. If you really believe that the task will improve your IBS symptoms, you will be more likely to follow through with it. Do research or meet with your health care providers if you need to clear up any concerns or doubts you have about a planned task.

Austin set a goal of sticking to his plan for the next year. He decided to keep a copy of his plan in his desk drawer at work and on his bedside table at home. Every Tuesday, either at work or at home, he would patiently take the time to read over his plan and make any necessary changes. Once a month he would make a date with a friend for a game of racket ball as a reward for sticking to the plan.

Plan for Possible Problems

Anticipate that you will run into roadblocks in any plan you make. Problem solve and find other options. For example, there will be periods such as holidays or busy times at work when you will have time crunches. If you plan for these in advance, you can adjust your plan accordingly. For example, you may need to cut back on your longer relaxation exercises for a few days and do more frequent mini-relaxation exercises.

Collin, a study participant, was a grant writer for a group of small nonprofit companies. He had a plan that managed his symptoms effectively— most of the time. When a big deadline approached, he found that he was getting less sleep and struggling to eat small, frequent meals and that his automatic thoughts were problems. For Collin, jumping to conclusions and overgeneralization specifically led to feelings of anxiety and dread. His symptoms increased, and he struggled painfully through each day.

When Collin completed his grant, he knew he had to add something to his plan. He decided to write an additional plan specific to the stresses of grant deadlines. He decided that a week before a deadline, he would eliminate all possible trigger foods, including coffee, and take a week's worth of snacks to the office to increase the possibility of eating small, frequent meals. He would begin and end his day with a few minutes of abdominal breathing and try to stretch or do a mini-relaxation exercise every hour during the day. After each meal, he would take a few minutes to review his thinking, looking for automatic thoughts that lead to feelings of anxiety. He would remind himself that he always gets his grants in on time. There is no reason to think that this one would not be on time also.

Collin tried this plan for the next grant. It did help decrease his symptoms but not as much as he hoped. With the next grant, he decided that he would begin 2 days earlier, giving himself more time to complete the research and begin the writing. He hoped that beginning earlier would also allow him to get at least 7 hours of sleep a night the week before the grant was due. Eventually, Collin began to see an improvement in his symptoms even when he was facing major deadlines at work.

Keep a Positive, Forgiving Attitude

You can encourage or discourage yourself by the way you talk and think. If you fail to meet a goal or complete a task, try to figure out what got in the way, problem solve, and then just get back to business. Give yourself positive suggestions and encouragement. Believing that you can stick to your plan creates the positive mental attitude needed to make changes.

Katie was the mother of three children, two sons in middle school and a daughter in high school. She found that her ability to stick to her plan fluctuated with her children's schedules. As they were finishing up each quarter in school, their school responsibilities increased as did their extracurricular activities. Her children were up later with homework, projects, sports, and rehearsals. As they got busier, she got busier. She had less time to complete all of the strategies that helped her manage her symptoms. With her new cognitive skills, Katie knew that blaming her children or herself for this lapse would only increase feelings that aggravate her symptoms.

So, Katie decided that she would just accept this as a part of the ebb and flow of life. There were times when she was too busy to get everything done. But those times passed, and she believed in her ability to get back to following her plan. She focused on doing as much as was possible each day and letting the rest go. After all, even a little is better than none. She was surprised to see that this system worked well. She had a mild increase in her symptoms at the end of each school period but not enough of an increase that she struggled to keep up with the needs of her children.

Be Flexible

It is important to include flexibility in your plan. If it's too rigid, it sets you up for discouragement and failure. Go back and review your plan if it isn't working. You may need to find a different way to approach your goal. For example, if you can't find a place to be alone to do relaxation exercises at work, you may need to take a walk at lunchtime instead. Either way, it addresses the same goals: to reduce stress and increase relaxation.

Abby began walking 4 times a week when she was in the IBS study. Walking was an effective way for her to relax and wind down after a busy day at work. She walked for a month, enjoying being out of doors before she went home to start dinner for her family. When fall arrived and the days got shorter, Abby began finding reasons to skip her walk. By the middle of October, she wasn't walking at all. Although her symptoms hadn't increased noticeably, she was aware that she felt less relaxed and was more irritable at work and with the kids.

Abby approached the lack of exercise in a new way. Instead of using all-or-nothing thinking or labeling, she reminded herself that many people exercise less in the fall and winter. Looking into alternatives, she found a gym near her home that would fit the budget and her schedule. She began stopping on the way home from work to exercise. The return of exercise helped her feel more relaxed and less irritable.

Relapses

Expect relapses. IBS symptoms are episodic and will show up from time to time. It is important to remember that by getting back on your comprehensive plan, you can get your symptoms back under control, often in just a few days.

If you do have a relapse, use the Keeping Track form to record your symptoms and identify the causes. Problem solve to see what strategy would be most helpful in this situation. Then write down a plan of action to get back on track. Remember that being successful at doing something always takes more than one try.

Resources

We hope this book will continue to be a resource for you in managing your IBS symptoms. It is a good idea to reread it periodically as a reminder of the strategies you found most helpful. Now that you are more experienced with stress, diet, and thought management, you may be able to learn and use exercises that were difficult for you when you were just beginning.

Most people who put the time and energy into learning and practicing the strategies in this book found that their symptoms improved. In earlier studies, we discovered that symptoms continue to improve for several months after participants completed the study. Many told us that, although they still had IBS, it no longer ruled their life. That is mastering it! As others walked through difficult times in their lives, they told us that they were thankful they didn't have to deal with IBS symptoms on top of everything else. And still others told us they found that this program affected many areas of their lives: their IBS was better and they were able to live a life that was rich and satisfying, enjoying children, grandchildren, travel, jobs, school, hobbies, and entertainment.

It has been a joy to walk alongside these study participants. They have worked hard and gained control over their symptoms. We wish the same for you also.

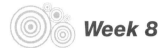 ***Week 8***

Skills to Build

Planning

Using the form provided in this chapter, write a comprehensive plan to manage your IBS symptoms. Include the strategies that you have found to be most helpful.

Self-Awareness

Complete the Keeping Track form each day until your plan is complete and working for you.

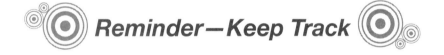

Common IBS Medications

Treating Symptoms with Medicine

We have presented multiple effective ways to manage your IBS symptoms in this book. If you practice these strategies regularly, you will greatly reduce your need for medications to treat IBS symptoms.

No medication exists that cures IBS. However, several prescribed or over-the-counter medications can improve specific symptoms of IBS, primarily abdominal pain, constipation, diarrhea, and gas. Because most medications are aimed at improving only one IBS symptom, you may end up using a combination of medications in your treatment.

Listed below are the most common symptoms of IBS and the medicines that are generally recommended for treatment.

Abdominal Pain

Antispasmodics are most commonly used to treat abdominal pain and bloating (Table 9). They have the potential to relieve bloating and cramping by reducing the frequency and intensity of smooth muscle spasms in the intestine. Antispasmodics are best taken 30 minutes before meals or as ordered to reduce pain.

Antidepressants are used for treatment of chronic pain associated with IBS. Antidepressants work to regulate neurotransmitters, the chemicals in the nervous system that send messages by stimulating the cells. The most common types of antidepressants used for treating IBS are selective serotonin reuptake inhibitors (SSRIs) and tricyclic antidepressants (TCAs).

Table 9. Antispasmodics for Abdominal Pain and Bloating

Brand Name	Generic Name	Common Side Effects
Librax	Chlordiazepoxide + clidinium bromide	Headaches, dizziness, blurred vision, dry mouth, difficulty emptying bladder, decreased sweating, nasal congestion, stuffiness, rash or itching, and constipation
Bentyl	Dicyclomine	
Levsin, Levbid, Levision Timecaps	Hycoscyamine sulfate	

Research has shown that, for some people, small doses of SSRIs or TCAs help decrease pain by increasing the level of serotonin, a hormone found in both the gut and the brain. At higher doses, these drugs are used to treat depression. Common brand names of SSRIs are Prozac, Paxil, Zoloft, Celexa, and Lexapro. Common generic (brand) names of SSRIs are fluoxetine (Prozac), paroxetine (Paxil), sertraline (Zoloft), citalopram (Celexa), and escitalopram (Lexapro). Common brand names of TCAs are imipramine (Tofranil), amitriptyline (Elavil), desipramine (Norpramin), clomipramine (Anafranil), and nortriptyline (Pamelor). The most common side effects associated with SSRIs include nausea, headaches, insomnia, and sexual dysfunction. Some common side effects associated with TCAs include dry mouth, blurred vision, constipation, nausea, difficulty urinating, drowsiness, and rapid heartbeat.

Pain relievers such as acetaminophen (Tylenol) and aspirin are sufficient to relieve the dull discomfort that can be part of the IBS symptom pattern. Avoid using opiates or narcotics, such as Tylenol with codeine, oxycodone, or vicodin, for pain management. These medications can make your IBS symptoms worse because of their impact on the intestine. For people with IBS who have stomach pain, antacids such as Maalox, Mylanta, and Tums can help ease the discomfort.

Constipation

As addressed in Chapter 6, the treatment of choice for constipation-prone IBS is dietary fiber. If you continue to have problems with constipation after carefully and slowly increasing your daily dietary fiber, you might try fiber supplements taken at mealtimes.

Soluble fiber, which dissolves in water to form a gel such as Metamucil or Konsyl, or a semisynthetic fiber such as Citrucel are available without a prescription. An insoluble synthetic fiber, which is not changed by the digestive system, such as FiberCon is also available for purchase. All synthetic fiber products may cause increased intestinal gas.

Lubiprostone (Amitiza) is a drug that can be beneficial for treating constipation in IBS. Products containing polyethylene glycol (PEG), although not specifically designed to treat IBS, may also help relieve constipation. Miralax and Glycolax are two such drugs.

Diarrhea

Lomotil is an antidiarrheal drug available by prescription only. It works by blocking acetylcholine, a hormone that increases the rhythmic contractions of the intestines. This drug should only be taken for up to 48 hours and may cause constipation.

Other antidiarrheal drugs that don't require a prescription include Pepto-Bismol and loperamide (Imodium). Pepto-Bismol helps stimulate absorption of fluids and electrolytes across the intestinal wall. Loperamide is commonly recommended to decrease stool frequency and improve stool consistency. It acts by slowing down movement of intestines and increases water absorption but may not reduce abdominal pain or distention. Talk with your health care provider to find the appropriate antidiarrheal agent for you to use.

Gas

Gas can result as normal bacteria in the large intestine digest complex carbohydrates from starches, fiber, and sugars. Beano is an over-the-counter, oral enzyme that helps break down complex carbohydrates in cruciferous vegetables and beans, decreasing the amount of gas produced.

Gas-X, Mylanta Gas, and Maalox Anti-Gas are all brand names of simethicone and are also available without a prescription. Simethicone is used to relieve symptoms of too much gas in the stomach or intestines. It works by dispersing the gas in the intestine and preventing it from collecting in pockets.

A combination of chlordiazepoxide and clidinium bromide (brand name Librax) can be helpful for those with excessive bloating.

IBS-Specific Medications

Only one medication is approved by the U.S. Food and Drug Administration (FDA) for the management of IBS symptoms. Alosetron (Lotronex) has been found to be effective for women with diarrhea-predominant IBS. However, due to serious and unpredictable adverse events, including some that resulted in deaths, the drug was withdrawn from the market in November 2000. In July 2002, the drug was put back on the market, but with a restricted distribution and use program: it is only for treatment of women with severe diarrhea-predominant IBS who have failed to respond to conventional treatment, and it can only be prescribed by physicians who are enrolled in a risk-management program offered by the drug manufacturer. These physicians must agree to educate patients on the risks and benefits of alosetron and provide patients with a copy of the FDA-approved medication guide. Patients are also asked to read and sign a patient-physician agreement before receiving their initial prescription for alosetron.

Guidelines for Medications

Don't over rely on medications to control your IBS symptoms. Long-term use of medications that may help decrease symptoms of IBS can potentially damage your gut and aggravate symptoms. Therefore, it's best to manage your IBS symptoms by using the self-management techniques you have found to be most effective.

Keep a medicine record. Write down each medicine you take, including over-the-counter medications, herbal preparations, and naturopathic remedies. Be sure to include the reason you take the medication or supplement, the dosage, and how often and the time of day you take it.

Tell your health care provider about any prescribed medication, over-the-counter medications, herbal preparations, or naturopathic remedies you are taking.

Ask your health care provider the following questions about any pre-scribed medications:

- What is the name of the medicine? Is this the brand name or generic name? Does it matter which one is used?
- What is the medicine supposed to do?
- How and when should it be taken?
- What foods, drinks, or other medications should be avoided while taking this medicine?
- What are the possible side effects? What do I do if they occur?
- Is there any written information about the medicine?[1]

[1]From *Prescription Medicines and You.* AHCPR Publication No. 96-0056, October 1999. Agency for Health Care Policy and Research and the National Council on Patient Information and Education, Rockville, MD, and Washington, DC. http://www.ahrp.goc/consumer/ncpiebro.htm

Extra Forms

Keeping Track Form

Circle the average level of discomfort you experienced for each symptom over the past 24 hours: 0, none; 1, mild; 2, moderate; 3, severe. Use the left column to write your goals for this week.

DATE							
Abdominal pain	3 2 1 0	3 2 1 0	3 2 1 0	3 2 1 0	3 2 1 0	3 2 1 0	3 2 1 0
Diarrhea	3 2 1 0	3 2 1 0	3 2 1 0	3 2 1 0	3 2 1 0	3 2 1 0	3 2 1 0
Constipation	3 2 1 0	3 2 1 0	3 2 1 0	3 2 1 0	3 2 1 0	3 2 1 0	3 2 1 0
Bloating	3 2 1 0	3 2 1 0	3 2 1 0	3 2 1 0	3 2 1 0	3 2 1 0	3 2 1 0
Stress	3 2 1 0	3 2 1 0	3 2 1 0	3 2 1 0	3 2 1 0	3 2 1 0	3 2 1 0
My goals this week:							
	Yes No #___	Yes No #___	Yes No #___	Yes No #___	Yes No #___	Yes No #___	Yes No #___
	Yes No #___	Yes No #___	Yes No #___	Yes No #___	Yes No #___	Yes No #___	Yes No #___
	Yes No #___	Yes No #___	Yes No #___	Yes No #___	Yes No #___	Yes No #___	Yes No #___
	Yes No #___	Yes No #___	Yes No #___	Yes No #___	Yes No #___	Yes No #___	Yes No #___

Keeping Track Form

Circle the average level of discomfort you experienced for each symptom over the past 24 hours: 0, none; 1, mild; 2, moderate; 3, severe. Use the left column to write your goals for this week.

DATE							
Abdominal pain	3 2 1 0	3 2 1 0	3 2 1 0	3 2 1 0	3 2 1 0	3 2 1 0	3 2 1 0
Diarrhea	3 2 1 0	3 2 1 0	3 2 1 0	3 2 1 0	3 2 1 0	3 2 1 0	3 2 1 0
Constipation	3 2 1 0	3 2 1 0	3 2 1 0	3 2 1 0	3 2 1 0	3 2 1 0	3 2 1 0
Bloating	3 2 1 0	3 2 1 0	3 2 1 0	3 2 1 0	3 2 1 0	3 2 1 0	3 2 1 0
Stress	3 2 1 0	3 2 1 0	3 2 1 0	3 2 1 0	3 2 1 0	3 2 1 0	3 2 1 0
My goals this week:							
	Yes No #___	Yes No #___	Yes No #___	Yes No #___	Yes No #___	Yes No #___	Yes No #___
	Yes No #___	Yes No #___	Yes No #___	Yes No #___	Yes No #___	Yes No #___	Yes No #___
	Yes No #___	Yes No #___	Yes No #___	Yes No #___	Yes No #___	Yes No #___	Yes No #___
	Yes No #___	Yes No #___	Yes No #___	Yes No #___	Yes No #___	Yes No #___	Yes No #___

Keeping Track Form

Circle the average level of discomfort you experienced for each symptom over the past 24 hours: 0, none; 1, mild; 2, moderate; 3, severe. Use the left column to write your goals for this week.

DATE							
Abdominal pain	3 2 1 0	3 2 1 0	3 2 1 0	3 2 1 0	3 2 1 0	3 2 1 0	3 2 1 0
Diarrhea	3 2 1 0	3 2 1 0	3 2 1 0	3 2 1 0	3 2 1 0	3 2 1 0	3 2 1 0
Constipation	3 2 1 0	3 2 1 0	3 2 1 0	3 2 1 0	3 2 1 0	3 2 1 0	3 2 1 0
Bloating	3 2 1 0	3 2 1 0	3 2 1 0	3 2 1 0	3 2 1 0	3 2 1 0	3 2 1 0
Stress	3 2 1 0	3 2 1 0	3 2 1 0	3 2 1 0	3 2 1 0	3 2 1 0	3 2 1 0
My goals this week:							
	Yes No #___	Yes No #___	Yes No #___	Yes No #___	Yes No #___	Yes No #___	Yes No #___
	Yes No #___	Yes No #___	Yes No #___	Yes No #___	Yes No #___	Yes No #___	Yes No #___
	Yes No #___	Yes No #___	Yes No #___	Yes No #___	Yes No #___	Yes No #___	Yes No #___
	Yes No #___	Yes No #___	Yes No #___	Yes No #___	Yes No #___	Yes No #___	Yes No #___

Keeping Track Form

Circle the average level of discomfort you experienced for each symptom over the past 24 hours: 0, none; 1, mild; 2, moderate; 3, severe. Use the left column to write your goals for this week.

DATE							
Abdominal pain	3 2 1 0	3 2 1 0	3 2 1 0	3 2 1 0	3 2 1 0	3 2 1 0	3 2 1 0
Diarrhea	3 2 1 0	3 2 1 0	3 2 1 0	3 2 1 0	3 2 1 0	3 2 1 0	3 2 1 0
Constipation	3 2 1 0	3 2 1 0	3 2 1 0	3 2 1 0	3 2 1 0	3 2 1 0	3 2 1 0
Bloating	3 2 1 0	3 2 1 0	3 2 1 0	3 2 1 0	3 2 1 0	3 2 1 0	3 2 1 0
Stress	3 2 1 0	3 2 1 0	3 2 1 0	3 2 1 0	3 2 1 0	3 2 1 0	3 2 1 0
My goals this week:							
	Yes No #___	Yes No #___	Yes No #___	Yes No #___	Yes No #___	Yes No #___	Yes No #___
	Yes No #___	Yes No #___	Yes No #___	Yes No #___	Yes No #___	Yes No #___	Yes No #___
	Yes No #___	Yes No #___	Yes No #___	Yes No #___	Yes No #___	Yes No #___	Yes No #___
	Yes No #___	Yes No #___	Yes No #___	Yes No #___	Yes No #___	Yes No #___	Yes No #___

Keeping Track Form

Circle the average level of discomfort you experienced for each symptom over the past 24 hours: 0, none; 1, mild; 2, moderate; 3, severe. Use the left column to write your goals for this week.

DATE							
Abdominal pain	3 2 1 0	3 2 1 0	3 2 1 0	3 2 1 0	3 2 1 0	3 2 1 0	3 2 1 0
Diarrhea	3 2 1 0	3 2 1 0	3 2 1 0	3 2 1 0	3 2 1 0	3 2 1 0	3 2 1 0
Constipation	3 2 1 0	3 2 1 0	3 2 1 0	3 2 1 0	3 2 1 0	3 2 1 0	3 2 1 0
Bloating	3 2 1 0	3 2 1 0	3 2 1 0	3 2 1 0	3 2 1 0	3 2 1 0	3 2 1 0
Stress	3 2 1 0	3 2 1 0	3 2 1 0	3 2 1 0	3 2 1 0	3 2 1 0	3 2 1 0
My goals this week:							
	Yes No #___	Yes No #___	Yes No #___	Yes No #___	Yes No #___	Yes No #___	Yes No #___
	Yes No #___	Yes No #___	Yes No #___	Yes No #___	Yes No #___	Yes No #___	Yes No #___
	Yes No #___	Yes No #___	Yes No #___	Yes No #___	Yes No #___	Yes No #___	Yes No #___
	Yes No #___	Yes No #___	Yes No #___	Yes No #___	Yes No #___	Yes No #___	Yes No #___

Keeping Track Form

Circle the average level of discomfort you experienced for each symptom over the past 24 hours: 0, none; 1, mild; 2, moderate; 3, severe. Use the left column to write your goals for this week.

DATE							
Abdominal pain	3 2 1 0	3 2 1 0	3 2 1 0	3 2 1 0	3 2 1 0	3 2 1 0	3 2 1 0
Diarrhea	3 2 1 0	3 2 1 0	3 2 1 0	3 2 1 0	3 2 1 0	3 2 1 0	3 2 1 0
Constipation	3 2 1 0	3 2 1 0	3 2 1 0	3 2 1 0	3 2 1 0	3 2 1 0	3 2 1 0
Bloating	3 2 1 0	3 2 1 0	3 2 1 0	3 2 1 0	3 2 1 0	3 2 1 0	3 2 1 0
Stress	3 2 1 0	3 2 1 0	3 2 1 0	3 2 1 0	3 2 1 0	3 2 1 0	3 2 1 0
My goals this week:							
	Yes No #___	Yes No #___	Yes No #___	Yes No #___	Yes No #___	Yes No #___	Yes No #___
	Yes No #___	Yes No #___	Yes No #___	Yes No #___	Yes No #___	Yes No #___	Yes No #___
	Yes No #___	Yes No #___	Yes No #___	Yes No #___	Yes No #___	Yes No #___	Yes No #___
	Yes No #___	Yes No #___	Yes No #___	Yes No #___	Yes No #___	Yes No #___	Yes No #___

Keeping Track Form

Circle the average level of discomfort you experienced for each symptom over the past 24 hours: 0, none; 1, mild; 2, moderate; 3, severe. Use the left column to write your goals for this week.

DATE							
Abdominal pain	3 2 1 0	3 2 1 0	3 2 1 0	3 2 1 0	3 2 1 0	3 2 1 0	3 2 1 0
Diarrhea	3 2 1 0	3 2 1 0	3 2 1 0	3 2 1 0	3 2 1 0	3 2 1 0	3 2 1 0
Constipation	3 2 1 0	3 2 1 0	3 2 1 0	3 2 1 0	3 2 1 0	3 2 1 0	3 2 1 0
Bloating	3 2 1 0	3 2 1 0	3 2 1 0	3 2 1 0	3 2 1 0	3 2 1 0	3 2 1 0
Stress	3 2 1 0	3 2 1 0	3 2 1 0	3 2 1 0	3 2 1 0	3 2 1 0	3 2 1 0
My goals this week:							
	Yes No #___	Yes No #___	Yes No #___	Yes No #___	Yes No #___	Yes No #___	Yes No #___
	Yes No #___	Yes No #___	Yes No #___	Yes No #___	Yes No #___	Yes No #___	Yes No #___
	Yes No #___	Yes No #___	Yes No #___	Yes No #___	Yes No #___	Yes No #___	Yes No #___
	Yes No #___	Yes No #___	Yes No #___	Yes No #___	Yes No #___	Yes No #___	Yes No #___

Keeping Track Form

Circle the average level of discomfort you experienced for each symptom over the past 24 hours: 0, none; 1, mild; 2, moderate; 3, severe. Use the left column to write your goals for this week.

DATE							
Abdominal pain	3 2 1 0	3 2 1 0	3 2 1 0	3 2 1 0	3 2 1 0	3 2 1 0	3 2 1 0
Diarrhea	3 2 1 0	3 2 1 0	3 2 1 0	3 2 1 0	3 2 1 0	3 2 1 0	3 2 1 0
Constipation	3 2 1 0	3 2 1 0	3 2 1 0	3 2 1 0	3 2 1 0	3 2 1 0	3 2 1 0
Bloating	3 2 1 0	3 2 1 0	3 2 1 0	3 2 1 0	3 2 1 0	3 2 1 0	3 2 1 0
Stress	3 2 1 0	3 2 1 0	3 2 1 0	3 2 1 0	3 2 1 0	3 2 1 0	3 2 1 0
My goals this week:							
	Yes No #___	Yes No #___	Yes No #___	Yes No #___	Yes No #___	Yes No #___	Yes No #___
	Yes No #___	Yes No #___	Yes No #___	Yes No #___	Yes No #___	Yes No #___	Yes No #___
	Yes No #___	Yes No #___	Yes No #___	Yes No #___	Yes No #___	Yes No #___	Yes No #___
	Yes No #___	Yes No #___	Yes No #___	Yes No #___	Yes No #___	Yes No #___	Yes No #___

Food Journal

Date: _____

Time	Symptoms	Stress level	Food	Fiber

Fruit (☐ ☐ ☐ ☐) ☐ ☐ Vegetables (☐ ☐ ☐ ☐ ☐) ☐ ☐ ☐ Grains (☐ ☐ ☐ ☐ ☐ ☐) ☐ ☐ ☐ ☐
Dairy (☐ ☐ ☐) ☐ ☐ Meats and Beans ☐ ☐ ☐ ☐ ☐ ☐ 8 oz. of water ☐ ☐ ☐ ☐ ☐ ☐ ☐ ☐
Symptoms: P, abdominal pain or cramping; D, diarrhea; C, constipation; B, bloating.
Rate pain and stress: 1 = mild; 2 = moderate; 3 = severe.

Food Journal

Date: _____

Time	Symptoms	Stress level	Food	Fiber

Fruit (☐ ☐ ☐ ☐) ☐ ☐ Vegetables (☐ ☐ ☐ ☐ ☐) ☐ ☐ ☐ Grains (☐ ☐ ☐ ☐ ☐ ☐) ☐ ☐ ☐ ☐
Dairy (☐ ☐ ☐) ☐ ☐ Meats and Beans ☐ ☐ ☐ ☐ ☐ ☐ 8 oz. of water ☐ ☐ ☐ ☐ ☐ ☐ ☐ ☐
Symptoms: P, abdominal pain or cramping; D, diarrhea; C, constipation; B, bloating.
Rate pain and stress: 1 = mild; 2 = moderate; 3 = severe.

Food Journal

Date: _____

Time	Symptoms	Stress level	Food	Fiber

Fruit (☐ ☐ ☐ ☐) ☐ ☐ Vegetables (☐ ☐ ☐ ☐ ☐) ☐ ☐ ☐ Grains (☐ ☐ ☐ ☐ ☐ ☐) ☐ ☐ ☐ ☐
Dairy (☐ ☐ ☐) ☐ ☐ Meats and Beans ☐ ☐ ☐ ☐ ☐ ☐ 8 oz. of water ☐ ☐ ☐ ☐ ☐ ☐ ☐ ☐
Symptoms: P, abdominal pain or cramping; D, diarrhea; C, constipation; B, bloating.
Rate pain and stress: 1 = mild; 2 = moderate; 3 = severe.

Food Journal

Date: _____

Time	Symptoms	Stress level	Food	Fiber

Fruit (☐ ☐ ☐ ☐) ☐ ☐ Vegetables (☐ ☐ ☐ ☐ ☐) ☐ ☐ ☐ Grains (☐ ☐ ☐ ☐ ☐ ☐) ☐ ☐ ☐ ☐
Dairy (☐ ☐ ☐) ☐ ☐ Meats and Beans ☐ ☐ ☐ ☐ ☐ ☐ 8 oz. of water ☐ ☐ ☐ ☐ ☐ ☐ ☐ ☐
Symptoms: P, abdominal pain or cramping; D, diarrhea; C, constipation; B, bloating.
Rate pain and stress: 1 = mild; 2 = moderate; 3 = severe.

Food Journal

Date: _____

Time	Symptoms	Stress level	Food	Fiber

Fruit (☐ ☐ ☐) ☐ ☐ Vegetables (☐ ☐ ☐ ☐) ☐ ☐ ☐ Grains (☐ ☐ ☐ ☐ ☐) ☐ ☐ ☐ ☐
Dairy (☐ ☐ ☐) ☐ ☐ Meats and Beans ☐ ☐ ☐ ☐ ☐ 8 oz. of water ☐ ☐ ☐ ☐ ☐ ☐ ☐ ☐
Symptoms: P, abdominal pain or cramping; D, diarrhea; C, constipation; B, bloating.
Rate pain and stress: 1 = mild; 2 = moderate; 3 = severe.

Food Journal

Date: _____

Time	Symptoms	Stress level	Food	Fiber

Fruit (☐ ☐ ☐ ☐) ☐ ☐ Vegetables (☐ ☐ ☐ ☐ ☐) ☐ ☐ ☐ Grains (☐ ☐ ☐ ☐ ☐ ☐) ☐ ☐ ☐ ☐
Dairy (☐ ☐ ☐) ☐ ☐ Meats and Beans ☐ ☐ ☐ ☐ ☐ ☐ 8 oz. of water ☐ ☐ ☐ ☐ ☐ ☐ ☐ ☐
Symptoms: P, abdominal pain or cramping; D, diarrhea; C, constipation; B, bloating.
Rate pain and stress: 1 = mild; 2 = moderate; 3 = severe.

Food Journal

Date: _____

Time	Symptoms	Stress level	Food	Fiber

Fruit (☐ ☐ ☐ ☐) ☐ ☐ Vegetables (☐ ☐ ☐ ☐ ☐) ☐ ☐ ☐ Grains (☐ ☐ ☐ ☐ ☐ ☐) ☐ ☐ ☐ ☐
Dairy (☐ ☐ ☐) ☐ ☐ Meats and Beans ☐ ☐ ☐ ☐ ☐ ☐ 8 oz. of water ☐ ☐ ☐ ☐ ☐ ☐ ☐ ☐
Symptoms: P, abdominal pain or cramping; D, diarrhea; C, constipation; B, bloating.
Rate pain and stress: 1 = mild; 2 = moderate; 3 = severe.

Food Journal

Date: _____

Time	Symptoms	Stress level	Food	Fiber

Fruit (☐ ☐ ☐ ☐) ☐ ☐ Vegetables (☐ ☐ ☐ ☐ ☐) ☐ ☐ ☐ Grains (☐ ☐ ☐ ☐ ☐ ☐) ☐ ☐ ☐ ☐
Dairy (☐ ☐ ☐) ☐ ☐ Meats and Beans ☐ ☐ ☐ ☐ ☐ ☐ 8 oz. of water ☐ ☐ ☐ ☐ ☐ ☐ ☐ ☐
Symptoms: P, abdominal pain or cramping; D, diarrhea; C, constipation; B, bloating.
Rate pain and stress: 1 = mild; 2 = moderate; 3 = severe.

Trigger Foods List

Food	Notes
Dairy	
Milk	
Yogurt	
Ice cream	
Cheese	
Cottage cheese	
Sour cream	
Vegetables	
Broccoli	
Cauliflower	
Cabbage	
Brussels sprouts	
Onions	
Corn	
Peas	
Potatoes	
Fruit	
Apples	
Pears	
Citrus fruit	
Bananas	
Berries	

Trigger Foods List (*Continued*)

Food	Notes
Meats/Beans/Nuts	
Eggs	
Pinto beans	
Kidney beans	
Lentils	
High-fat red meat	
Nuts	
Breads/Cereal	
Wheat	
Miscellaneous	
Humus	
Garlic	
Coffee	
Chocolate	
Beer	
Wine (white or red)	
Liquor	
Sorbitol	
Spicy foods	
High-fat foods	
Other	

Trigger Foods List

Food	Notes
Dairy	
Milk	
Yogurt	
Ice cream	
Cheese	
Cottage cheese	
Sour cream	
Vegetables	
Broccoli	
Cauliflower	
Cabbage	
Brussels sprouts	
Onions	
Corn	
Peas	
Potatoes	
Fruit	
Apples	
Pears	
Citrus fruit	
Bananas	
Berries	

Trigger Foods List (*Continued*)

Food	Notes
Meats/Beans/Nuts	
Eggs	
Pinto beans	
Kidney beans	
Lentils	
High-fat red meat	
Nuts	
Breads/Cereal	
Wheat	
Miscellaneous	
Humus	
Garlic	
Coffee	
Chocolate	
Beer	
Wine (white or red)	
Liquor	
Sorbitol	
Spicy foods	
High-fat foods	
Other	

My Action Plan

1. This week I will:

When will I do this?

What obstacles might keep me from reaching my goal?

How can I overcome these obstacles?

2. This week I will:

When will I do this?

What obstacles might keep me from reaching my goals?

How can I overcome these obstacles?

My Action Plan

1. This week I will:

When will I do this?

What obstacles might keep me from reaching my goal?

How can I overcome these obstacles?

2. This week I will:

When will I do this?

What obstacles might keep me from reaching my goals?

How can I overcome these obstacles?

My Action Plan

1. This week I will:

When will I do this?

What obstacles might keep me from reaching my goal?

How can I overcome these obstacles?

2. This week I will:

When will I do this?

What obstacles might keep me from reaching my goals?

How can I overcome these obstacles?

My Action Plan

1. This week I will:

When will I do this?

What obstacles might keep me from reaching my goal?

How can I overcome these obstacles?

2. This week I will:

When will I do this?

What obstacles might keep me from reaching my goals?

How can I overcome these obstacles?

My Action Plan

1. This week I will:

When will I do this?

What obstacles might keep me from reaching my goal?

How can I overcome these obstacles?

2. This week I will:

When will I do this?

What obstacles might keep me from reaching my goals?

How can I overcome these obstacles?

My Action Plan

1. This week I will:

When will I do this?

What obstacles might keep me from reaching my goal?

How can I overcome these obstacles?

2. This week I will:

When will I do this?

What obstacles might keep me from reaching my goals?

How can I overcome these obstacles?

Automatic Thoughts Form

Event →	Thoughts →	Feelings →	Behavior/symptoms

Automatic Thoughts Form

Event →	Thoughts →	Feelings →	Behavior/symptoms

Automatic Thoughts Form

Event →	Thoughts →	Feelings →	Behavior/symptoms

Automatic Thoughts Form

Event →	Thoughts →	Feelings →	Behavior/symptoms

Automatic Thoughts Form

Event →	Thoughts →	Feelings →	Behavior/symptoms

Automatic Thoughts Form

Event →	Thoughts →	Feelings →	Behavior/symptoms

Problem-Solving Worksheet

1. Define the problem. What is the goal of your problem solving? Be specific.

2. Brainstorm all possible solutions.

3. Evaluate each solution. Consider the pros and cons.

Possible Solutions	Pros	Cons

Problem-Solving Worksheet (*Continued*)

4. Pick the best solution. List specific steps you need to take to put the solution into action.

5. Put the solution into action.

6. Evaluate the results. Modify the solution or return to step one if you are not satisfied.

Problem-Solving Worksheet

1. Define the problem. What is the goal of your problem solving? Be specific.

2. Brainstorm all possible solutions.

3. Evaluate each solution. Consider the pros and cons.

Possible Solutions	Pros	Cons

Problem-Solving Worksheet (*Continued*)

4. Pick the best solution. List specific steps you need to take to put the solution into action.

5. Put the solution into action.

6. Evaluate the results. Modify the solution or return to step one if you are not satisfied.

Problem-Solving Worksheet

1. Define the problem. What is the goal of your problem solving? Be specific.

2. Brainstorm all possible solutions.

3. Evaluate each solution. Consider the pros and cons.

Possible Solutions	Pros	Cons

Problem-Solving Worksheet (*Continued*)

4. Pick the best solution. List specific steps you need to take to put the solution into action.

5. Put the solution into action.

6. Evaluate the results. Modify the solution or return to step one if you are not satisfied.

Problem-Solving Worksheet

1. Define the problem. What is the goal of your problem solving? Be specific.

2. Brainstorm all possible solutions.

3. Evaluate each solution. Consider the pros and cons.

Possible Solutions	Pros	Cons

Problem-Solving Worksheet (*Continued*)

4. Pick the best solution. List specific steps you need to take to put the solution into action.

5. Put the solution into action.

6. Evaluate the results. Modify the solution or return to step one if you are not satisfied.

Problem-Solving Worksheet

1. Define the problem. What is the goal of your problem solving? Be specific.

2. Brainstorm all possible solutions.

3. Evaluate each solution. Consider the pros and cons.

Possible Solutions	Pros	Cons

Problem-Solving Worksheet (*Continued*)

4. Pick the best solution. List specific steps you need to take to put the solution into action.

5. Put the solution into action.

6. Evaluate the results. Modify the solution or return to step one if you are not satisfied.

Problem-Solving Worksheet

1. Define the problem. What is the goal of your problem solving? Be specific.

2. Brainstorm all possible solutions.

3. Evaluate each solution. Consider the pros and cons.

Possible Solutions	Pros	Cons

Problem-Solving Worksheet (*Continued*)

4. Pick the best solution. List specific steps you need to take to put the solution into action.

5. Put the solution into action.

6. Evaluate the results. Modify the solution or return to step one if you are not satisfied.

Steps for Correcting False Beliefs

Automatic thought:

Why does this bother me?

Why does that bother me?

Why does that bother me?

Why does that bother me?

False belief:

Is this belief true?

Does the belief serve me well at this point in my life?

How can I change the belief to make it more accurate and useful?

New accurate belief:

Steps for Correcting False Beliefs

Automatic thought:

Why does this bother me?

Why does that bother me?

Why does that bother me?

Why does that bother me?

False belief:

Is this belief true?

Does the belief serve me well at this point in my life?

How can I change the belief to make it more accurate and useful?

New accurate belief:

Steps for Correcting False Beliefs

Automatic thought:

Why does this bother me?

Why does that bother me?

Why does that bother me?

Why does that bother me?

False belief:

Is this belief true?

Does the belief serve me well at this point in my life?

How can I change the belief to make it more accurate and useful?

New accurate belief:

Steps for Correcting False Beliefs

Automatic thought:

Why does this bother me?

Why does that bother me?

Why does that bother me?

Why does that bother me?

False belief:

Is this belief true?

Does the belief serve me well at this point in my life?

How can I change the belief to make it more accurate and useful?

New accurate belief:

Steps for Correcting False Beliefs

Automatic thought:

Why does this bother me?

Why does that bother me?

Why does that bother me?

Why does that bother me?

False belief:

Is this belief true?

Does the belief serve me well at this point in my life?

How can I change the belief to make it more accurate and useful?

New accurate belief:

Steps for Correcting False Beliefs

Automatic thought:

Why does this bother me?

Why does that bother me?

Why does that bother me?

Why does that bother me?

False belief:

Is this belief true?

Does the belief serve me well at this point in my life?

How can I change the belief to make it more accurate and useful?

New accurate belief:

My Pain Management Plan

My IBS symptoms generally occur:

The early cues for these symptom are:
Thoughts:

Feelings:

Physical sensations:

Actions to reduce or relieve these symptoms:
Diet:

Thoughts:

Relaxation:

My Pain Management Plan

My IBS symptoms generally occur:

The early cues for these symptom are:
Thoughts:

Feelings:

Physical sensations:

Actions to reduce or relieve these symptoms:
Diet:

Thoughts:

Relaxation:

My Pain Management Plan

My IBS symptoms generally occur:

The early cues for these symptom are:
Thoughts:

Feelings:

Physical sensations:

Actions to reduce or relieve these symptoms:
Diet:

Thoughts:

Relaxation:

My Pain Management Plan

My IBS symptoms generally occur:

The early cues for these symptom are:
Thoughts:

Feelings:

Physical sensations:

Actions to reduce or relieve these symptoms:
Diet:

Thoughts:

Relaxation:

My Pain Management Plan

My IBS symptoms generally occur:

The early cues for these symptom are:
Thoughts:

Feelings:

Physical sensations:

Actions to reduce or relieve these symptoms:
Diet:

Thoughts:

Relaxation:

My Pain Management Plan

My IBS symptoms generally occur:

The early cues for these symptom are:
<u>Thoughts</u>:

<u>Feelings</u>:

<u>Physical sensations</u>:

Actions to reduce or relieve these symptoms:
<u>Diet</u>:

<u>Thoughts</u>:

<u>Relaxation</u>:

Sleep Diary

Day number and date	Last night I went to bed at:	Last night I fell asleep at:	Number of times I woke up during the night	I got up at:	Number of hours that I slept	When I awoke, I felt: (circle one)	My sleep was disturbed by: (mental, emotional, physical, or environmental factors)
Day 1 date	am/pm	am/pm	# of times	am/pm	hours	Refreshed Somewhat refreshed Fatigued	
Day 2 date	am/pm	am/pm	# of times	am/pm	hours	Refreshed Somewhat refreshed Fatigued	
Day 3 date	am/pm	am/pm	# of times	am/pm	hours	Refreshed Somewhat refreshed Fatigued	
Day 4 date	am/pm	am/pm	# of times	am/pm	hours	Refreshed Somewhat refreshed Fatigued	
Day 5 date	am/pm	am/pm	# of times	am/pm	hours	Refreshed Somewhat refreshed Fatigued	
Day 6 date	am/pm	am/pm	# of times	am/pm	hours	Refreshed Somewhat refreshed Fatigued	
Day 7 date	am/pm	am/pm	# of times	am/pm	hours	Refreshed Somewhat refreshed Fatigued	

Sleep Diary

Day number and date	Last night I went to bed at:	Last night I fell asleep at:	Number of times I woke up during the night	I got up at:	Number of hours that I slept	When I awoke, I felt: (circle one)	My sleep was disturbed by: (mental, emotional, physical, or environmental factors)
Day 1 date	 am/pm	 am/pm	 # of times	 am/pm	 hours	Refreshed Somewhat refreshed Fatigued	
Day 2 date	 am/pm	 am/pm	 # of times	 am/pm	 hours	Refreshed Somewhat refreshed Fatigued	
Day 3 date	 am/pm	 am/pm	 # of times	 am/pm	 hours	Refreshed Somewhat refreshed Fatigued	
Day 4 date	 am/pm	 am/pm	 # of times	 am/pm	 hours	Refreshed Somewhat refreshed Fatigued	
Day 5 date	 am/pm	 am/pm	 # of times	 am/pm	 hours	Refreshed Somewhat refreshed Fatigued	
Day 6 date	 am/pm	 am/pm	 # of times	 am/pm	 hours	Refreshed Somewhat refreshed Fatigued	
Day 7 date	 am/pm	 am/pm	 # of times	 am/pm	 hours	Refreshed Somewhat refreshed Fatigued	

Sleep Diary

Day number and date	Last night I went to bed at:	Last night I fell asleep at:	Number of times I woke up during the night	I got up at:	Number of hours that I slept	When I awoke, I felt: (circle one)	My sleep was disturbed by: (mental, emotional, physical, or environmental factors)
Day 1 date	am/pm	am/pm	# of times	am/pm	hours	Refreshed Somewhat refreshed Fatigued	
Day 2 date	am/pm	am/pm	# of times	am/pm	hours	Refreshed Somewhat refreshed Fatigued	
Day 3 date	am/pm	am/pm	# of times	am/pm	hours	Refreshed Somewhat refreshed Fatigued	
Day 4 date	am/pm	am/pm	# of times	am/pm	hours	Refreshed Somewhat refreshed Fatigued	
Day 5 date	am/pm	am/pm	# of times	am/pm	hours	Refreshed Somewhat refreshed Fatigued	
Day 6 date	am/pm	am/pm	# of times	am/pm	hours	Refreshed Somewhat refreshed Fatigued	
Day 7 date	am/pm	am/pm	# of times	am/pm	hours	Refreshed Somewhat refreshed Fatigued	

Sleep Diary

Day number and date	Last night I went to bed at:	Last night I fell asleep at:	Number of times I woke up during the night	I got up at:	Number of hours that I slept	When I awoke, I felt: (circle one)	My sleep was disturbed by: (mental, emotional, physical, or environmental factors)
Day 1 date	am/pm	am/pm	# of times	am/pm	hours	Refreshed Somewhat refreshed Fatigued	
Day 2 date	am/pm	am/pm	# of times	am/pm	hours	Refreshed Somewhat refreshed Fatigued	
Day 3 date	am/pm	am/pm	# of times	am/pm	hours	Refreshed Somewhat refreshed Fatigued	
Day 4 date	am/pm	am/pm	# of times	am/pm	hours	Refreshed Somewhat refreshed Fatigued	
Day 5 date	am/pm	am/pm	# of times	am/pm	hours	Refreshed Somewhat refreshed Fatigued	
Day 6 date	am/pm	am/pm	# of times	am/pm	hours	Refreshed Somewhat refreshed Fatigued	
Day 7 date	am/pm	am/pm	# of times	am/pm	hours	Refreshed Somewhat refreshed Fatigued	

Sleep Diary

Day number and date	Last night I went to bed at:	Last night I fell asleep at:	Number of times I woke up during the night	I got up at:	Number of hours that I slept	When I awoke, I felt: (circle one)	My sleep was disturbed by: (mental, emotional, physical, or environmental factors)
Day 1 date	am/pm	am/pm	# of times	am/pm	hours	Refreshed Somewhat refreshed Fatigued	
Day 2 date	am/pm	am/pm	# of times	am/pm	hours	Refreshed Somewhat refreshed Fatigued	
Day 3 date	am/pm	am/pm	# of times	am/pm	hours	Refreshed Somewhat refreshed Fatigued	
Day 4 date	am/pm	am/pm	# of times	am/pm	hours	Refreshed Somewhat refreshed Fatigued	
Day 5 date	am/pm	am/pm	# of times	am/pm	hours	Refreshed Somewhat refreshed Fatigued	
Day 6 date	am/pm	am/pm	# of times	am/pm	hours	Refreshed Somewhat refreshed Fatigued	
Day 7 date	am/pm	am/pm	# of times	am/pm	hours	Refreshed Somewhat refreshed Fatigued	

Sleep Diary

Day number and date	Last night I went to bed at:	Last night I fell asleep at:	Number of times I woke up during the night	I got up at:	Number of hours that I slept	When I awoke, I felt: (circle one)	My sleep was disturbed by: (mental, emotional, physical, or environmental factors)
Day 1 date	am/pm	am/pm	# of times	am/pm	hours	Refreshed Somewhat refreshed Fatigued	
Day 2 date	am/pm	am/pm	# of times	am/pm	hours	Refreshed Somewhat refreshed Fatigued	
Day 3 date	am/pm	am/pm	# of times	am/pm	hours	Refreshed Somewhat refreshed Fatigued	
Day 4 date	am/pm	am/pm	# of times	am/pm	hours	Refreshed Somewhat refreshed Fatigued	
Day 5 date	am/pm	am/pm	# of times	am/pm	hours	Refreshed Somewhat refreshed Fatigued	
Day 6 date	am/pm	am/pm	# of times	am/pm	hours	Refreshed Somewhat refreshed Fatigued	
Day 7 date	am/pm	am/pm	# of times	am/pm	hours	Refreshed Somewhat refreshed Fatigued	